Understanding Patient Safety

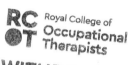

Understanding Patient Safety

edited by
Lynne Currie

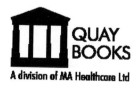

QUAY
BOOKS
A division of MA Healthcare Ltd

Quay Books Division, MA Healthcare Ltd, St Jude's Church, Dulwich Road, London SE24 0PB

British Library Cataloguing-in-Publication Data
A catalogue record is available for this book

© MA Healthcare Limited 2007
ISBN-10: 1-85642-289-5
ISBN-13: 978-1-85642-289-5

Printed in the UK by Athenaeum Press Ltd, Dukesway, Team Valley, Gateshead, NE11 0PZ

CONTENTS

Note

Health care practice and knowledge are constantly changing and developing as new research and treatments, changes in procedures, drugs and equipment become available.

The author and publishers have, as far as is possible, taken care to confirm that the information complies with the latest standards of practice and legislation.

LIST OF CONTRIBUTORS

Jane Carthey, Safety Improvement Specialist, National Patient Safety Agency

Lynne Currie, Project Manager: Evaluating and Improving, Royal College of Nursing Institute, Oxford

Philomena Fox, Clinical Risk Manager, Nottingham City Hospitals NHS Trust, Nottingham

Wendy Harris, Head of Safety Solutions, National Patient Safety Agency

Annette Jeanes, Consultant Nurse Infection Control and Director of Infection Prevention University College London Hospitals Foundation Trust

Peter Mansell, Director for Patient Experience, National Patient Safety Agency

Frank Milligan, Lecturer in Nursing Practice, Faculty of Health and Social Sciences, University of Bedfordshire

Cherrill Scott, Senior Research fellow, Royal College of Nursing Institute, London

Ross Scrivener, Programme Manager: Online Resources, Royal College of Nursing Institute, London

Imran Haider Syed, Research Associate, National Patient Safety Agency

Susan Watt, Education and Clinical Effectiveness Adviser, Royal College of Nursing, Scotland

Elizabeth West, Director of Research, School of Health and Social Care, University of Greenwich, London

FOREWORD

Seven years after the publication of *An Organisation with a Memory* patient safety has become a global priority for healthcare. Between 2000 and the present time there has been a proliferation of developments in the UK National Health Service (NHS), not least the establishment of the National Patient Safety Agency (NPSA) and the National Reporting and Learning System (NRLS), which is the first national reporting system in the world. We can be justly proud of these developments.

The title of this book encapsulates its purpose. We hope that on reading this book you will begin to see the importance of building a safer healthcare system that keeps patients safe from accidental harm. As our healthcare system becomes increasingly more complex, this complexity makes it likely that opportunities for error will continue to proliferate. Improving patient safety requires a concerted effort by government, professional organisations, healthcare regulators, professionals, policy makers and consumers. It becomes ever more important to ensure that tribal boundaries between professions are overcome, and any remnants of a culture of blame be disassembled. Organisations need to be better at reporting failures in patient safety, and continuously demonstrate their ability to learn from past mistakes. Patients and the general public will expect no less.

We hope this book will appeal to a wide range of readers that includes healthcare professionals, patients and the wider general public. Chapter 1 provides the context in which patient safety has become an international priority, and includes an overview of the role of the media, a description of key terms and definitions; an outline of key policy initiatives, and a discussion on the impact organisational silence has on patient safety. Chapter 2 outlines the importance attached to engendering a culture of safety across the NHS and outlines the differences between safety culture and safety climate. Through a series of case studies Chapter 3 explores the professional, organisational and bureaucratic inadequacies that have led to breakdowns in patient safety. Chapter 4 outlines the context in which greater patient and publication participation has been instrumental in shaping the work of the NPSA. Chapter 5 considers the impact of nursing staffing shortages on patient safety through an examination of the research evidence. Chapter 6 highlights some of the national imperatives that are driving the way healthcare organisations manage risk. Chapter 7 outlines the background to, and principles of infection control, and describes the actions required by organisations, patients and the general public. Chapter 8 considers the range of patient safety resources currently available via the Internet, and offers readers a number of ways to navigate the rapidly expanding information highway.

However, no single book can fully hope to cover an area as diverse as patient safety. As this book goes to press new books and journal articles abound on the many diverse elements of patient safety. Anyone whose interest in patient safety has been stimulated by reading this book is directed to read some of the seminal works that are referenced, and search out the wealth of material that is being produced by people who are committed to improving the safety of patients across the world.

Lynne Currie
Project Manager: Evaluating and Improving, Royal College of
Nursing Institute, Oxford

CHAPTER 1

An Introduction to Patient Safety

Lynne Currie, Susan Watt

'More people die in a given year as a result of medical errors than from motor vehicle accidents...breast cancer....or AIDS'

Institute of Medicine, 2000: 1

Healthcare, we are told, is a risky and increasingly complex business. However, the idea of keeping patients safe throughout their illness experience underpins the very essence of healthcare, and is grounded in the Hippocratic Oath to '*do no harm*'. The concept of 'patient safety' has gained prominence over the last decade or so, with concerted efforts to improve patient safety emphasising the need to ensure that patients, wherever they receive care and treatment, are kept safe from unintended injuries, accidental injuries, or harm. The emphasis on unintended injury or unintended harm is crucial, and is premised on a belief that no one working in healthcare sets out to deliberately harm a patient.

There are of course some exceptions to this (Shipman Report, 2004), however the vast majority of healthcare workers do their very best to ensure all patients are kept safe from harm. Failures in patient safety occur as a result of organisational system failures, or what are sometimes referred to as (unintended) errors, and these are the subject of this chapter. The issues surrounding cases of intentional or malicious harm are expanded in chapter three.

This chapter begins by providing the background or context in which patient safety came to be seen as an international priority for healthcare. It includes an overview of the influential role of the media in providing added impetus in the drive to improve patient safety across the world, considers the implications arising as a result of key patient safety failures in the United Kingdom (UK), and provides a description of some of key terms and definitions around patient safety. The chapter then moves to a discussion of the key policy initiatives pertaining to patient safety, including a description of the number of errors occurring in the NHS, and how these errors are, or are not reported, before describing a range of methods used to investigate patient safety failures. The chapter also provides a synopsis of a wide range of patient safety research initiatives and the ethics of disclosing errors, before culminating in a discussion around organisational silence and its impact on patient safety.

Background

The first concerted emphasis on patient safety occurred in Australia in 1987 with the establishment of the Australian Patient Safety Foundation (Runciman, 2002). This in turn led to the creation of the Australian Incident Monitoring System (AIMS), which was the worlds' first voluntary, anonymous national reporting system. The purpose of a national reporting system is fivefold:

- Collect information from a range of sources
- Be just
- Separate the processes for accountability from the processes of learning
- Provide feedback and information about action plans
- Involve and inform patients, public and professionals.

More recently, both the World Health Organisation (WHO) and the European Union (EU) have grasped the nettle of patient safety with the launch of the Patient Safety Alliance (WHO, 2004), and the Luxembourg Declaration on Patient Safety (European Commission, 2005).

Role of the Media

Over the last 15 years the media can be seen as being very influential in raising the profile of failures in patient safety in both the UK and the United States of America (USA). There is rising public concern over safety failures in health care, which have resulted in diminishing levels of public trust in healthcare professionals (Millenson, 2002). Whilst error rates are substantial, as will be discussed below, they are also perceived as being isolated and unusual events (Leape, 1994). Furthermore, a leading commentator in the field of patient safety has suggested that many in the medical professional remain in denial about the true scale of patient safety problems (Bagian, 2005). Bagian has argued that the failure to accept the numbers of patient safety failures ranges from:

> '...a lack of acceptance that a problem exists...[or] a combination in varying degrees of ignorance and arrogance'
>
> Bagian, 2005: 4

Patient safety developments in the USA came to the fore following the publication of an influential report (IOM, 1999), which estimated that large numbers of people die in hospitals each year as a result of preventable medial errors. These estimates were extrapolated from two large studies undertaken in US hospitals (Brennan et al, 1991). Although the problems surrounding patient safety in the USA have been highlighted in the medical literature since the 1950s, some have suggested that it was the public shaming of the medical professional in the US news media that forced the medical professional to address the issue of patient safety (Milenson, 2002). Some of the key patient safety failures that happened in the USA, which resulted in the media spotlight being turned on to healthcare, are graphically described by Millenson. They include the following:

- A female patient dying as a result of a massive overdose of a powerful anti-cancer drug
- The removal of the wrong breast during mastectomy
- A female patient dying as a result of her dialysis catheter being mistaken for a feeding tube
- A male patient dying as a result of his ventilator being mistakenly disconnected
- Arthroscopic surgery being undertaken on the wrong knee.

In the UK there have been a number of serious failures in the National Health Service (NHS) that have led to a sustained media interest in the way the NHS works, accompanied by a concerted policy drive towards improving patient safety. While the driver for the cultural transformation of the NHS was the events occurring at the Paediatric Cardiac Unit at the Bristol Royal Infirmary (Kennedy, 2001), other drivers include the actions of gynaecologist Rodney Ledward (Ritchie Report, 2000), and the retention of human organs and tissue following post mortem (Department of Health [DH], 2001a). The most recently publicised failure in the NHS is the case of Harold Shipman, but because his actions were clearly intentional this case is summarised in a later chapter.

Patient Safety Failures in the UK

The key messages from the Bristol Royal Infirmary scandal can be seen as the catalyst for major changes in the way patient safety is managed in the NHS. At the Paediatric Cardiac Unit located within the Bristol Royal Infirmary the absence of a culture of safety and openness resulted in concerns and incidents not being routinely or systematically discussed or addressed. This lack of openness and transparency compounded unsafe practice. There were also problems in both the physical environment of care and the working conditions which were identified as being just as important to patient safety as the technical skills of staff. The lack of systems at both national and local level for monitoring the safety of clinical care were said to put patients at increased risk, and the absence of any systematic approach to organisational learning resulted in the organisation's inability to learn the lessons from failure (Kennedy, 2001). Key importance is now attached to the idea that organisations must start to learn the lessons from failures, and there is a growing emphasis being placed on finding solutions to patient safety problems, which is discussed in more detail below.

During the evidence heard by the Bristol Inquiry it was also reported that the hearts of some of the children who had died had been removed during post-mortem examination. It was also noted that the practice of removing human organs following post-mortem had been going on in various hospitals over a period of 50 years. As a result of this, members of the public (in the main parents whose child had been given a post mortem) began to make enquiries across a range of hospitals and it transpired that large numbers of retained human organs and tissue were being stored in hospitals across the NHS (DH, 2001a). What angered parents was the practice of removing their child's organs and tissue without their knowledge or consent. This led the Chief Medical Officer to recommend that a code of practice should be instituted that would ensure required standards of communication with families about post-mortems (DH, 2001a).

The inquiry into the actions of gynaecologist Rodney Ledward made recommendations on a range of issues including incident reporting and whistle-blowing. The authors of the Ritchie Report defined clinical incident reporting as a system that aims to ensure that all untoward events occurring in hospital are identified and investigated and that lessons are learnt (Ritchie Report, 2000). In terms of whistle-blowing, the Ritchie Report notes that while a number of doctors were concerned about Rodney Ledward they reported feeling inhibited and unable to do anything about it because they did not want to be seen as telling tales. The authors of the report suggest that while a culture of not telling tales is powerful and superficially attractive, if care is to be truly patient-centred then all healthcare professionals have a duty to raise their concerns about colleagues with appropriate clinical or managerial staff. The Ritchie Report quotes the GMC Good Medical Practice booklet as saying that a doctor must:

> *'...protect patients when you believe that a doctor's or other colleague's health conduct or performance is a threat to them'*
>
> Ritchie Report, 2000

Put another way, this appears to suggest that it is the duty of healthcare professionals to always put the patient first, even if that means having to challenge their colleagues. However, a number of commentators have suggested that many healthcare professionals feel unable to voice their concerns about colleagues who do not practice safely (Millenson, 2005; Henriksen and Dayton, 2006). Recent research from the USA has identified the need for seven crucial conversations in healthcare in an effort to minimise the threat to patient safety as a result of organisational silence (Maxfield, et al, 2005).

This idea of organisational silence and its relationship to patient safety will be discussed in greater detail below.

UK Policy Context for Patient Safety

England and Wales

With greater attention now being paid to patient safety, and particular emphasis being placed on the levels of medical errors occurring in the NHS, the Government has formulated policy which is based on an understanding that such errors occur because of poorly designed systems. The whole tone of current policies on modernising the NHS is underpinned by the concept of cultural change, and the requirement to focus activities away from people towards an analysis of systems. Put another way, it is an attempt to move away from a culture of blame towards a culture of safety. The idea that organisation culture, and safety culture in particular, is a key determinant of the level at which patient safety is managed in NHS organisations is a key theme throughout this book and is discussed in greater depth in chapter 2.

While the UK Government continues to pursue policies aimed at ensuring the safety of all patients undergoing care and treatment in the NHS, the promotion of an effective patient safety agenda is a key priority of all the major health services across the world — the challenges faced are similar, with medication errors accounting for around a quarter of all incidents that threaten the safety of patients. It has also been suggested that there is a need for international standardisation of the terminology used to define and report medical errors, and there is said to be a will to collaborate in designing and implementing solutions for patient safety (Leatherman et al, 2000).

In outlining its plans for modernisation, the Government placed patient safety at the forefront of their commitment to quality, and established the need for a new national reporting system for error (DH, 2001b). In order to promote patient safety across England and Wales, the Government established the National Patient Safety Agency (NPSA) in July 2001. The NPSA is a Special Health Authority and has responsibility for developing a national reporting framework. Some of the innovative work being developed by the NPSA is described in chapter four. In all its policies on patient safety the UK Government has spelled out its commitment to embed a culture of safety across all NHS treatment (DH, 2004), the importance of which is discussed in greater detail in chapter two.

Northern Ireland

Northern Ireland Executive's first Programme for Government in 2001 included a commitment to raise the quality and safety of public services. A Ministerial agreement to proposals in the consultation document '*Best Practice Best Care*', published by the Department of Health, Social Services and Public Safety (DHSSPS, 2001) meant that for the first time the Health and Personal Social Services (HPSS) organisations had to fulfil a statutory duty of safety and quality (DHSSPS, 2001). In 2003 a legal framework for quality of health and social services was created through the HPSS Quality, Improvement and Regulation (Northern Ireland) Order 2003, which also extended quality improvement to a wider group of services.

Since March 2005, the National Clinical Assessment Service (NCAS) and NPSA have provided services to the NHS in Northern Ireland, under a service level agreement with the DHSSPS. In April 2005, the DHSSPS established the Regulation and Quality Improvement Authority (RQIA) as a non departmental public body with its independence guaranteed in law. The RQIA encourages improvements in the standards of health and social care provision through reporting and feedback of the findings of their reviews. All care facilities in Northern Ireland must register with the RQIA, and all care homes are inspected annually.

The RQIA monitor care provision through a review system using '*Clinical and Social Care Governance*', and they examine standards and how well the service is provided by looking at what went wrong and ways of making sure it does not happen again. The RQIA make recommendations to the service provider and offer a range of safety solutions that are derived from the lessons learned from failure (RQIA, 2006).

Scotland

The strategic direction for health care in Scotland is outlined in *Delivery for Health* (Scottish Executive, 2005a) and *Building a Health Service Fit for the Future* (Scottish Executive, 2005b). Guidance on implementing the objectives outlined in these policy documents has been issued to the NHS in Scotland and is underpinned by a number of key themes, including patient safety, patient experience, and quality improvement. In addition to a commitment to deliver improved health outcomes, the Scottish Executive has reviewed progress towards these objectives against six dimensions of quality (IOM, 2001) and improving patient safety has been identified as a priority area for further development.

NHS Quality Improvement Scotland (NHS QIS) was established in January 2003, bringing together a number of organisations involved in patient safety, clinical effectiveness and quality improvement. Its role is to improve the quality of health care in Scotland through setting standards, monitoring performance, providing guidance and advice, and supporting NHS Boards to deliver continuous improvements in patient safety.

The Clinical Governance and Patient Safety Support Unit (CGPSSU), established in 2004, is tasked with drawing together existing guidance and best practice to establish and consolidate patient safety improvements across Scotland. Taking a patient-centred approach is at the heart of all NHS activity in Scotland, and it is an approach that is underpinned by a principle of learning from experience to ensure that all care delivered to patients in Scotland, wherever they live, is safe, effective and of good quality.

Definitions and Terminology

There are a number of definitions currently in use, and some of the most commonly found terms are described.

'Patient safety' is defined as freedom from accidental injury, medical error, or an adverse event (Mohr et al, 2004).

'Accidental injury' or *'medical error'* is defined as the failure of a planned action to be completed as intended or the use of a wrong plan to achieve an aim (Mohr, et al, 2004).

An *'adverse event'* is defined as any incident whereby a patient is harmed by their care or treatment (Mohr et al, 2004). More recently the term being used by the NPSA is *'patient safety incident'* which is defined as any incident which may lead to a patient being harmed (NPSA, 2003). This definition clearly includes the idea of a 'near miss'.

A *'near miss'* is viewed as any unintended or unexpected incident which could have potentially harmed a patient but was recovered before it did. The key importance of identifying and reporting near misses is linked to the way in which such practices help organisations learn lessons from potential failure through implementing actions plans to redesign the safety system.

Estimated Number of Patient Safety Failures in the NHS

Estimates regarding the numbers of patient deaths as a result of failures in patient safety in the NHS appear somewhat conflicting. The Department of Health (DH, 2000) puts the number of patient deaths at 400 a year, with 10,000 patients said to suffer a severe adverse reaction to drugs. Researchers have calculated that as many as 850,000 — which is roughly 10% of all NHS hospital admissions — suffer a patient safety incident (Vincent et al, 2001). The same researchers suggest that the true scale of the problem remains unknown, and as yet the NHS has no data on how many patients receiving treatment in primary care suffer injury or death as a result of failures in patient safety.

The costs of preventable adverse events in the NHS have been calculated at £2b per annum, leading to an additional three million bed days (Vincent et al, 2001). More recent research has shown the number of patient deaths

Table 1.1. Estimated numbers of patient safety failures and near misses (Source: National Audit Office, 2005)

Number of patient safety failures and near misses reported in 2003–2004	855,832[1]
Number of patient safety failures and near misses reported in 2004–2005	974,000[2]
Number of patient deaths reported in 2004–2005	2,181[3]

Most common safety incidents reported:
- Patient injury due to falls
- Medication errors
- Equipment-related failures
- Documentation error
- Communication failure

[1] Few trusts included hospital acquired infections, which may increase the number by 300000–100000 of which may be preventable

[2] Under-reporting of near misses and patient safety failures costs the NHS £2bn per year and hospital acquired infections add a further £1bn per year

[3] Still significant levels of under-reporting suggest that as many as between 340–34000 patients die each year as a result of patient safety failures

to lie in the region of 40,000 (Health Foundation, 2004), whilst the National Patient Safety Agency (NPSA) comments that an extrapolation of research undertaken at two London hospitals would suggest as many as 72,000 patient deaths (NPSA, 2004).

However, more recent evidence suggests that from the numbers of patient safety incidents reported to the NRLS by 230 organisations, 1 in a 100 led to severe harm or death (NPSA, 2005). This report further suggests that while the estimated number of accidents is similar to the 850,000 quoted above, the number of deaths is considerably lower than 40,000. What one needs to bear in mind however, when interpreting these results is that the number of reports is by no means a definitive guide to the number of patient safety incidents that may actually occur in the NHS. This is because accident reporting is voluntary and confidential, and NHS organisations can choose to opt out of reporting to the NRLS.

A summary of the estimated number of patient safety incidents and near misses as reported by the National Audit Office (NAO, 2005) are shown in *Table 1.1*. The message to be taken from this is that we really do not know the extent and impact of patient safety incidents in the acute sector of the NHS, and we know even less about the levels occurring in the primary care sector.

Statistics from the Medical Defence Union (MDU) published in 1996 offers some indication of the level of medication errors occurring in general practice. The MDU reports that out of 790 claims settled, 25% of these were directly related to the prescribing, monitoring and administration of medicines, whilst 25 patient deaths were directly attributable to medical errors (Spink, 2004).

In the USA, commentators have calculated that between 44,000 and 98,000 hospitalised patients die annually as a result of medical error (IOM, 2000), with the number of deaths due to failures in safety exceeding that of deaths due to motor accidents, breast cancer and AIDS. Furthermore, this estimate of 98,000 excludes those patients who survive but who are left with serious injuries as a result. In Australia, estimates suggest that 16.6% of all patients admitted to hospital suffer an adverse event, 51.5% of which are preventable (Arah and Klazinga, 2004).

How to Investigate Failures in Patient Safety

There are two main approaches to the investigation of patient safety failure, or what is usually referred to as accidents or errors in the safety science literature (Reason, 1997, 2000; Reason et al, 2001).

The first is the person approach, which focuses on blame, and the second is the systems approach, which focuses on the chain of events leading up to an error. The person approach to error has been to focus on the actions of individual people and to blame them when things go wrong. This approach is underpinned by a belief that freedom from error is possible, and in the past this has been the approach most utilised when investigating errors in health care.

A system approach to error however is underpinned by a belief that people are fallible so we must expect errors to occur (Reason, 1997). Thus, errors happen because of poorly designed systems as opposed to poorly functioning human beings. The system approach to error is used widely in other industries including petrochemical, aviation, and nuclear energy, and is becoming increasingly talked about in health care.

There are two types of failure identified in the literature on safety (Vincent et al, 1998). An 'active failure' which is seen as an unsafe act or omission by someone whose actions can have an immediate effect, and a 'latent failure' which is seen as something that can lie dormant for years before combining with an active failure to cause an incident or an accident. Examples of active failures include giving the wrong medicine or removing the wrong kidney, whereas examples of latent failures include poor communication, ineffective leadership, inappropriate staffing levels and inadequate knowledge. Generally, active failures are said to occur at the 'sharp end' of care (the point of care delivery), whilst latent failures are said to occur at the 'blunt end' of care (management and administrative decision-making).

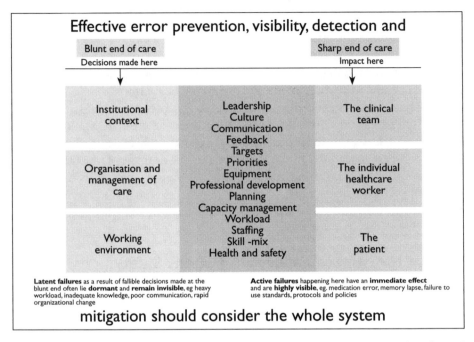

Figure 1.1. A holistic approach to the investigation of failures in patient safety (based on Nolan, 2000; Reason et al, 2001).

The elements at the sharp end of care have been described as the care team, the individual team member, the task, and the patient. The elements of the 'blunt end' are described as the institutional context, the organisation and management of care, and the work environment (Nolan, 2000). In addition there are said to be three key areas needed in the design of a safe system:

- Prevention (designing the system for safety)
- Visibility and detection (inspection, computerised prescribing, patient involvement and empowerment)
- Mitigation (learning the lessons, reforming the system) (Nolan, 2004).

Prevention, visibility and detection, and mitigation must be addressed at both the sharp and the blunt end of care delivery if patient safety is to be managed effectively (see *Figure 1.1* above). However, in the person approach to error described above it is possible to see how a continued emphasis on individual blame keeps things very firmly within the sharp end of the care continuum.

There is a belief that latent failures are generated at those working at the blunt end of care, for example decision-makers, managers and equipment designers, whilst active failures occurring at the sharp end of care are usually associated with the performance of front line clinical staff, for example, doctors, nurses other healthcare workers (Busse and Wright, 2000).

Tools for Investigating Patient Safety Failures

Root Cause Analysis

The NPSA have chosen to focus on Root Cause Analysis (RCA) as the way to investigate patient safety failures. RCA is advocated on the premise that it is a mechanism by which errors and near misses can be investigated, and it signifies an attempt to get at the 'root' of a problem (Carroll et al, 2002). It usually involves a multi-professional team asking three questions of an event:

- What happened?
- Why did it happen?
- What can be done to prevent it happening again?
  (Gosbee and Anderson, 2002).

However, RCA is by definition reactive rather than proactive because it explores the reasons for errors that have already occurred.

Some commentators suggest that RCA teams may focus on a breach of policies and procedures and an individual's personal shortcomings, rather than focusing on systemic factors (Busse and Wright, 2000). RCA has the potential to continue to blame individuals when things go wrong. Others have argued that while RCA is currently the most advocated form of retrospective review, it is not clearly defined and its implementation is variable (Hofer and Hayward, 2002). While the purpose of RCA is to uncover all the causes of an error including any underlying organisational factors from isolated case reports, in reality this is difficult. In addition, RCA is can be very expensive to undertake, it can take a long time, it may fail to establish why things went wrong, and it may also fail to guarantee any improvements in redesigning systems for safety. However, RCA does have its champions who argue that it shows promise, and that it is not the tool *per se* that is important — it is the institutional context in which the tool is introduced and used. Put another way, what may be more crucial than the tool used to investigate the causes of error is the type of culture that is present in an organisation at the time the error occurred (Carroll et al, 2002).

Hazard Analysis and Critical Control Point/Failure, Model and Effect Analysis

An alternative to RCA is Hazard Analysis and Critical Control Point (HACCP), which has been used in managing food safety in the NHS (Wilson et al, 1997). This model of proactive incident analysis was developed in the USA by Pilsbury and

Table 1.2. Principles of hazard analysis critical control point (HACCP) (Source: Food and Agriculture Organisation of the United Nations)

Principle 1   Conduct a hazard analysis (identify hazards and assess all associated risks and describe all possible control measures

Principle 2   Determine the critical control point (CCP)[1]

Principle 3   Establish critical limits[2]

Principle 4   Establish a monitoring system[3]

Principle 5   Establish a procedure for corrective action, when monitoring a CCP indicates a deviation from an established critical limit

Principle 6   Establish procedures for verification to confirm the effectiveness of the HACCP plan[4]

Principle 7   Establish appropriate documentation concerning all procedures and records

[1] A CCP is a step at which control can be applied and is essential to prevent or to eliminate a safety hazard, or reduce it to an acceptable level

[2] Each control measure associated with a CCP must have an associated critical limit which separates the acceptable from the unacceptable

[3] Monitoring is the scheduled measurement or observation at a CCP to assess whether the step is under control

[4] Such procedures include auditing the HACCP plan to review deviations, and random sampling and checking to validate the whole plan

Table 1.3. Steps in proactively evaluating a healthcare process (Source: De Posier et al, 2002)

Step 1   Define the topic[1]

Step 2   Assemble the team[2]

Step 3   Graphically describe the process[3]

Step 4   Conduct a hazard analysis[4]

Step 5   Actions and outcomes measures[5]

[1] This should be a high-risk or high-vulnerability area to warrant the investment of time and resources

[2] The team should be multidisciplinary and include subject experts, an advisor and a team leader

[3] Develop and verify the process flow diagram and consecutively number each step in the process

[4] List all possible/potential failure modes for each of the sub-processes and consecutively number these failure modes

[5] Develop a description of action for each failure mode cause, identity outcome measures, and identify one person responsible for completing or for ensuring the completion of each action

NASA and is based on the engineering system Failure, Mode and Effect Analysis (FMEA). It is underpinned by seven principles and is used to explore the potential for things to go wrong at critical points (See *Table 1.2*). At the time of writing this chapter no literature outlining the use of HACCP in the area of patient safety in the NHS was found. However, it may be that the seven principles outlined in *Table 1.2* could be developed for use in clinical practice, either as an algorithm, an integrated care pathway, or through the use of clinical audit. The principles of HACCP and FMEA have been adapted for use in the USA, and a tutorial is available outlining five key steps in proactively evaluating a health care process (See *Table 1.3*).

Unreported Patient Safety Failures

I have discussed above the conflicting information about the numbers of patient safety failures in health care. Elsewhere it has been cogently argued that failures go under-reported for a number of reasons: a lack of awareness of the severity of the problem; a belief that most errors do no harm to patients; and the perception that it is difficult to deal with human error when it does happen (Leape, 1994). Furthermore, it has also been suggested that people do not report errors because they do not think it will make any difference, or they are scared of reporting theirs or their colleagues' errors because they are afraid of being seen as careless or of speaking out of turn (Leape, 2000). Indeed, there is anecdotal evidence to suggest that very often it is those reporting the error that are scapegoated and made to feel so uncomfortable that they have to leave the organisation — as was the case for the anaesthetist who blew the whistle on what was happening at the Bristol Royal Infirmary, who emigrated to Australia.

A recent report on the current state of patient safety in the NHS revealed that while many NHS Trusts in the acute sector have developed a more just and fair culture there are still some organisations who continue to operate a blame culture thus inhibiting incident reporting (NAO, 2005). The five main reasons for failing to report patient safety incidents and near misses are summarised in *Table 1.4*, some of which may be related to the culture that operates across an organisation.

There is also a sense that healthcare professionals are socialised, through their education and training into believing they should not make errors. It may be that this notion of invulnerability compounds all efforts to increase reporting and publicly disclose safety failures. This socialisation process is described as a culture in which making a mistake is clearly linked with an individual's moral failing, thus encouraging denial (Ottewill, 2003), and it actually reinforces the attachment to the person approach to error described above. The challenge according to Bagian is the need to get:

> *'...all healthcare personnel to acknowledge that, given the right set of circumstances, any individual or institution can harm a patient. Getting past*

> ### Table 1.4. Main reasons for failing to report patient safety incidents and near misses (Source: National Audit Office, 2005)
>
> - Fear
> - Poorly designed forms
> - Lack of understanding about what to report
> - Failure to recognise that an incident (or near miss) has occurred
> - Being too busy
> - Lack of feedback

this individual and organisational form of denial is critical if any progress is to be made.... [and] individuals who believe that safety is not an issue for them individually are viewed as the most dangerous person in the room'

Bagian, 2005: 6

However, I would go further and suggest that it is also crucial that patients and the general public are made more aware of the fact that humans make mistakes, and in this respect healthcare professionals are no different from the rest of us. We need to understand that just because someone makes an error this does not mean they are incompetent neither does it mean they are bad person. It is also important to clarify that what often infuriates people who experience problems in their health care is that when they approach organisations and professionals in seeking information about what has gone wrong they often face intransigence, a lack of empathy and a failure to acknowledge that a problem has occurred.

Patient Safety Research

The Professional and Policymakers' View of Patient Safety
The bulk of research investigating patient safety issues is primarily policy and professionally driven, with much research focusing on medication error, which is an area of high risk, and as reported above is said to account for 20% of patient safety incidents.

There are a number of ways in which a medication error can occur, including: giving the wrong drug to the right patient; giving the right drug to the wrong patient; giving the drug at the wrong time; or not giving the drug at all. In addition, a medical error can also occur when a drug is given by the wrong route, as for example giving a drug intrathecally (into the spine) when it should have been given intravenously (through the vein). However, too exclusive a focus on how medicines are administered, whilst important, may mask problems associated with prescribing errors, illegible handwriting (Osborne et al, 1999), or calculating the correct dosage (Gladstone, 1995).

Research has also highlighted that nurses (who are the professional group mostly likely to administer medicines) do get disciplined if they make a drug error (Firth-Cozens et al, 2001). However, prescribing errors made by doctors are not considered errors and often go unreported (Coles et al, 2001). While the true scale of prescribing errors in unknown, research in one London hospital found approximately that 135 were made each week, of which 34 were potentially serious. Whilst the majority of these errors originated in medication order writing, the most serious errors originated in the prescribing decision (Dean et al, 2002).

Another study examining the causes and consequences of safety failures cited the most common causes of error as job overload, inexperience, lack of supervision, and faulty judgement (Meurier et al, 1997). A literature review exploring the factors that contribute to medication errors (Meurier et al, 1997) suggested that these are the result of personnel, systems and managerial problems, all of which can be argued are latent failures occurring as a result of decisions that are made at the blunt end of care.

A more recent development in health care is new patient safety research being undertaken on what have been identified as the non-technical skills of healthcare professionals. Non-technical skills are said to complement the technical skills crucial in maintaining patient safety. These skills have been identified as teamwork, leadership, communication (interpersonal skills), decision-making, planning, situation awareness (cognitive skills) and they are said to complement technical skills (Flin and Yule, 2003; Yule et al, 2006) — see *Figure 1.2*.

Leadership skills mean having the ability to give direction in setting and maintaining high standards of safe clinical care, being able to cope with pressure, and being supportive and considerate about the needs of all team members. Teamwork and communication skills are exhibited through the ability to exchange relevant information and ensure that there is a shared understanding about that information across the team, as well as the ability to co-ordinate team activities. Being situationally aware requires an ability to gather and understand information and being able to project and anticipate where and when things might go wrong and taking action to prevent them going wrong. Effective decision-making relies on an ability to diagnose a situation and make a judgement about the most appropriate course of action. Effective planning skills are manifested in the way a person is able to organise resources, people and activities to achieve safety goals.

A key contributory factor in patient safety failures has been identified as poor communication (Donchin and Gopher, 2003; DH, 2001b). Research in the USA suggests that more than 60% of medication errors are due to failures in interpersonal communication (cited in Henrikson and Dayton, 2006). Linked

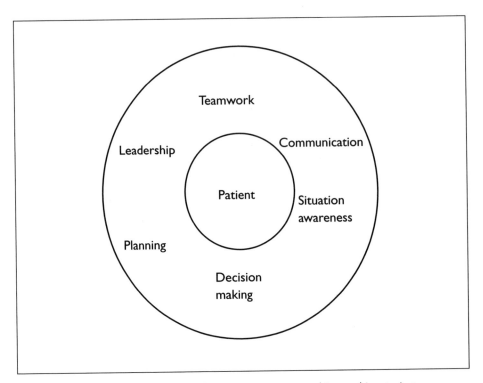

Figure 1.2. Key non-technical skills for improving partnership working to improve patient safety.

to this are the cultural barriers that often make it difficult for staff who witness errors to feel able to challenge their colleagues — as highlighted by the evidence put forward at the inquiries into Bristol (Kennedy, 2001) and the Ledward case (Ritchie Report, 2000). This may be especially congruent when a junior staff member faces challenging the decisions of a senior colleague, or when a nurse is faced with challenging a doctor.

While much of what is reported above focuses on medication error, which appears on the basis of what is described in the literature, to be the greatest threat to patient safety, there are many other potential sources of patient safety failures. These include the retention of instruments and sponges following surgery (Gwande, 2003), blood transfusion errors (SHOT, 2004), rising infection rates, self-harm (including suicide), use of restraints, incidence of pressure ulcers and slips, trips and falls. There is also a real need for research to explore how ordinary people think about patient safety, if only to see whether there is any convergence or divergence of opinion about what constitutes the greatest threat to patient safety — is it medication errors, or are there other things that might be equally important to patients?

Effective inter-professional teamwork has been identified as being crucial in the delivery of high quality safety patient care. It is dependent upon the non-technical skills as well as the technical proficiency of all members of the inter-professional team. Such teamwork is greatly facilitated in organisations that are said to have inculcated a culture of safety.

The Patients' View of Patient Safety

At present there appears to be limited literature on how patients understand the concept of patient safety. The National Patient Safety Foundation of the American Medical Association surveyed US households in order to understand the experiences and opinions of American adults on patient safety issues in health care (NPSF, 1997). Findings showed that while health care was felt to be moderately safe, it was viewed as being safer than nuclear power, and less safe than airline travel (NPSF, 1997). Up to 56% of respondents reported they had experience of being involved in a medical mistake, with 42% reporting being involved in more than one medical mistake. Furthermore, 29% of respondents suggested that carelessness or negligence on the part of healthcare professionals was the reason why medical mistakes happen (NPSF, 1997).

Research in France exploring 65 inpatients' knowledge and opinions about nosocomial infections found that while 17 of patients were able to describe them as hospital-acquired infections, 52 stated that during their time in hospital they had received no information about these types of infections. Furthermore, 33 patients said they would seek legal action against the hospital should they contract a nosocomial infection (Merle et al, 2005) .

Professional and Patient Views on the Disclosure of Error

Research has been undertaken to explore patients and professionals views of the need to disclosure medical errors. A study exploring both patients' and doctors' attitudes about medical error looked at whether doctors disclose the information patients want, the doctors' and patients' emotional needs when errors occur, and whether these needs were met (Gallagher et al, 2003). Findings suggest that both doctors and patients had unmet needs. Patients wanted full disclosure of harmful errors and sought information about what had happened, why it happened, and what would be done about it (Gallagher, et al, 2003). Doctors however, whilst agreeing that errors should be disclosed talked about how they would need to choose their words carefully when disclosing errors to patients. Doctors reported that when they did disclose an error they often avoided saying that an error had occurred, why it had occurred, and how it might be prevented. Patients reported that they wanted emotional support from doctors following errors, including an apology, whereas doctors felt that an apology would create legal liability (Gallagher et al, 2003). This idea that giving the patient an apology is an admittance of liability is false and has no legal basis, however, it is an idea that appears highly influential amongst some healthcare professionals.

A survey of Australian households on the anonymity and transparency of reporting medical error found that 94% of respondents believed that errors should be reported (Evans et al, 2004). Of those in favour of reporting (*n*=1856), 68% thought that healthcare workers should identify themselves, whilst 29.2% thought they should remain anonymous. The apparent public reluctance to accept anonymity and the confidential, voluntary nature of reporting (like the system we have in the NHS) may reflect some level of scepticism and a belief that the interests of both healthcare organisations and healthcare professionals are often placed above the interests of patients. Public preference certainly appears to be towards the individualising of error and perhaps some leaning towards apportioning blame when things go wrong. However, this is contrary to a quality improvement philosophy which promotes a system-based approach to error. Both the public and healthcare professionals need to be educated about the complexities of error and the vulnerability of both patients; and professionals (Evans et al, 2004). The findings from the Evans et al study resonate with earlier research undertaken in the USA, which reported that 62% of the public favoured the full public disclosure of errors, whilst 86% of doctors did not (Blendon et al, 2002).

Another survey examined the relationship between type of error, severity of outcome and the level of disclosure against five dependent variables:

- Likelihood of changing doctors
- Likelihood of seeking legal advice
- Patient satisfaction
- Trust
- Emotional response (Mazor et al, 2004).

In addition, the survey sought to determine patients' attitudes, beliefs and preferences about medical errors and disclosure in general. Findings suggest that full disclosure following a medical error reduces the likelihood that patients will change their doctor, and also results in a more positive emotional response. It may also reduce the likelihood that patients will seek legal advice in some, if not all circumstances.

Findings also suggest that doctors can influence the consequences of the disclosure process if they fully explain what happened, acknowledge responsibility, apologise, and ensure that steps will be taken to ensure the error does not happen again. Patients however, also reported being influenced by the severity of outcome and the specifics of the error situation, so doctors should not always assume that full disclosure will result in a positive response. Patients' said they wanted to be told about errors even if nothing can be done about them and that their own safety while being under the care of healthcare professionals is much more important to them than claiming compensation (Mazor et al, 2004).

The Ethics of Disclosure

From an ethical point of view the failure to tell a patient that an error has occurred not only undermines the public's trust in healthcare professionals because they may feel they are being deceived, but it also may appear to protect the professional rather than the patient. Professionals' codes of conduct are underpinned by a commitment to act solely for the patient's best interests, and the ability of patients to give informed consent to the treatment of an injury caused by medical error dictates that patients must be provided with all the relevant information pertaining to that error. Full disclosure of error is consistent with recent ethical advances in medicine towards openness and patient involvement in care, which involves informed consent and telling the truth.

At the heart of the ethical debate around the disclosure of errors is the principle that patients should be told about errors out of respect for them as persons, and that they have a right to know about errors — even if they have not been harmed. Furthermore, principles of justice and fairness demand that patients should be able to seek compensation if they have been injured as a result of medical error.

The rationale for full disclosure of error is based on the notion of autonomy. A belief that full disclosure will increase the patient's anxiety or serve to confuse the patient is patronising and serves once again to protect the professional. Furthermore, the non-disclosure of error undermines efforts to improve patient safety and reinforces non-reporting. Whilst the law recognises that healthcare professionals make mistakes, they still have both an ethical and a moral duty to inform the patient.

Organisational Silence

Staff ability or willingness to speak up about their safety concerns has been the subject of recent research in the USA (Maxfield et al, 2005) and the hidden threats to patient safety as a result of 'organisational silence' have been clearly described by Millenson (2003) and Henriksen and Dayton, 2006). Millenson takes particular issue with the apparent inability of healthcare professionals to confront their responsibility for patient safety. This inability he suggests is manifest in the silence of the deed — which he describes as a failure to take corrective action — and in the silence of the word — which is a failure to discuss openly the true consequences of their failure to act.

According to Millenson, many in the healthcare community: 'continue to avert their eyes....pay lip service to....improvement...' and believe that the problem 'is really about underpaid providers or meddling insurers or irresponsible patients' (Millenson, 2003: 103-104).

This apparent inability to take action against failures in patient safety over a considerable number of years has resulted in the preventable deaths of:

> *'...2.5 million men, women and children...in American hospitals between 1978 and 1999...[or if you]...divide the number of deaths by the average number of acute care hospitals during this period... what you end up with is 9 to 22 patients unnecessarily dying every year at every community hospital in the county, every year for 21 years...'*
>
> Millenson, 2003: 106

When we consider the scale of the events occurring at the Paediatric Unit of the Bristol Royal Infirmary during the period 1984–1995 and the number of women who were harmed by the actions of Rodney Ledward we can see how a culture of organisational silence operates to main the status-quo over a considerable number of years.

In expanding upon the concept of organisational silence, Henriksen and Dayton (2006) suggest that it refers to an organisations collective ability to say or do very little in response to the significant patient safety problems facing the healthcare industry today. This has also been referred to as 'cultural censorship' or 'consensual neglect'.

Cultural censorship has been invoked to describe the duplicitous nature of organisational life where patient safety failures paradoxically are both recognised and concealed, and where a lack of consensus about the causes of failure may provide a convenient cloak for assigning it to the expected risks of medical practice, and where implicit bonds of transgression are formed and become culturally acceptable with respect to questionable practices that are shared by providers as a way of getting things done. Fear of personal implication in the shared wrong doing or questionable practice serves to maintain the organisational silence" (Henrikson and Dayton, 2006). In relation to the Ledward affair we can see how:

> *'...the defining characteristics of cultural censorship can help us to understand how adverse events get pushed underground, only to flourish in the underside of organisational life'"*
>
> Hart and Hazelgrove, 2001: 257

The term 'consensual neglect' refers to the way in which decision-makers tend:

> *'...to tacitly ignore...unexpected events...in order to achieve unity of purpose and act as a single entity. Disruptive and politically incorrect issues are ignored, overly simplified, or become homogenised into more acceptable terms'"*
>
> Henrikson and Dayton, 2006: 1541

Table 1.5 Factors contributing to organisational silence and hidden threats to patient safety
(Source: Henrikson and Dayton, 2005)

FACTORS	ELEMENTS	DESCRIPTION
INDIVIDUAL	Availability heuristic	Due to the relatively small numbers of errors occurring in individual institutions many healthcare profession-als do not see the patient safety agenda as relevant to their organisation.
	Self-serving bias	When individuals do some-thing well they attribute their success to something in their disposition, and when they do something wrong they attribute their failure to a situation that is outside of their control.
	Status-quo trap	Organisational members show a clear tendency towards maintaining the status quo because this is more comfortable, requires no action and carries less psychological risk.
SOCIAL	Conformity	Organisational members adapt their judgements and beliefs to those around them in order to gain acceptance
	Diffusion of responsibility	Organisational members rend to take on less respon-sibility when efforts are pooled in achieving shared goals. Roles and responsibil-ities are assumed rather than being made explicit, and this leads to situations in which key elements of care may be missed, which can result in patient safety failures.
	Microclimates of mistrust	Organisational silence and under-reporting of error are likely to be manifest in local units, ward or departments where leaders tend to blame error on individual failings or incompetence. The style of leadership shapes and influ-ences the microclimate.

Continued on next page

ORGANISATIONAL	Unchallenged beliefs	There is a propensity for organisations to bring together highly qualified, expert groups and expect good decisions to emerge. Such groups sometimes reach consensus too quickly and dissenting voices may go unheard. Such groups display a tendency to 'group-think' leading them to focus only on information that confirms their initial beliefs and to disregard information that challenges those beliefs.
	The good provider fallacy	Whist most healthcare professionals hold a strong work ethic, and are highly committed, compassionate and resourceful, such quali-ties have an ironic dark side. Many professionals often employ quick fixes or first-order problem-solving when they see someone practising unsafely, and although such actions may satisfy immedi-ate patient needs they fail to address underlying causes and do not prevent the same things from happening time and again.
	Neglect of interdependencies	High levels of reliability and organisational learning are less likely to be realised when quick fix solutions are used to patch over process failures that either escape the attention of leaders or are tacitly condoned by them. Leaders are in a bet-ter position to address the causes of unsafe practices and remain mindful of the interdependencies of care, simply because they can work across organisational units and address any dis-continuities.

The authors go on to describe a number of less obvious threats that contribute to a culture of organisational silence, and these are summarised in *Table 1.5*.

A recent study in the USA found that while many healthcare workers witness their colleagues breaking rules, making mistakes, failing to offer support, appear to be incompetent, fail to work as part of a team, treat others disrespectfully and micromanage situations, less than 10% of them reported that they fail to do anything about it (Maxfield et al, 2005). Their reasons for doing nothing included lack of confidence, concerns over the effects of speaking up and fear of retaliation. The authors conclude that it is now critical that healthcare organisations create cultures of safety which enable healthcare professionals to speak out. The creation of such a culture would result in improvements in productivity, a reduction in nursing staff turnover and higher levels of cooperation from doctors. However, they also acknowledge that simply creating a culture of safety is not enough, and they recommended that leaders should make improving 'crucial conversations' their top priority (Maxfield, et al, 2005)

Conclusion

The challenge in reducing the number of patients who experience injury or even death as a result of medical error has been shown to be closely linked to a requirement to transform NHS culture, which is discussed in chapter two. Rhetoric exhorts that if NHS organisations can move from a culture of blame to one of justice and fairness, where safety is seen is paramount to all organisational activity, then they will be seen as having the wherewithal to reduce patient safety incidents that result from organisational system failures. However, the Corporate Manslaughter Act, which has received Royal Assent and comes into force from April 2008, creates an offence of corporate manslaughter in England, Wales and Northern Ireland, and corporate homicide in Scotland. Justice Minister Maria Eagle comments that:

'...this is a ground breaking piece of legislation. This is about ensuring justice for victims of corporate failures...We are sending a very powerful message to those organisations which do not take their health and safety responsibilities seriously'

Ministry of Justice, 2007

We can see that measures are in place to deal with the accountability of clinicians who are deemed to have been negligent (through the policies and procedures overseen by the General Medical Council and the Nursing and Midwifery Council). However in the past these mechanisms have failed patients whilst simultaneously protecting incompetent professionals and those who have acted with criminal intent. We need also to be reassured that there are robust mechanisms in place to ensure that senior managers and decision-makers are accountable for any serious shortcomings in the way their organisations manage patient safety.

All healthcare organisations need a clear, unequivocal focus on the goal of preventing harm to the patient, rather than an almost exclusive focus on eliminating error (Bagian, 2005), or an over emphasis on protecting the professional. In addition, there should be an explicit acknowledgement that it will never be possible to rid healthcare of error. The best that organisations can do is to ensure that all patient safety failures are reported and investigated, lessons are learned and shared, and that healthcare professionals and managers are held accountable for their actions and their decisions.

Taking a more pragmatic view, if organisations are to be seen as being successful in preventing harm to the patient there are a number of things that should happen. First, we should see a sharp increase in the levels of failures being reported across all sectors of healthcare. Second, we should expect to see more information being disclosed to the general public on the types and severity of patient safety failures, together with information on the steps that are being taken to address such failures. Third, we should expect to see more and more of this data becoming available through the NRLS leading to the identification of patterns or trends, and detailed information on patient safety solutions for the benefit of the whole health care system. Lastly we should start to see clear evidence that a culture of safety has been embedded throughout our healthcare system, one that is just and accountable and clearly differentiates the processes of accountability from the processes of learning.

As described above we are currently working on estimates of the number of hospitalised patients who suffer harm as a result of failures in patient safety, and we have little available data on failures across the primary and independent care sectors. While the most recent evidence from NRLS provides us with some data, the picture remains incomplete. However, any proliferation of data resulting from more open reporting of failure across the whole of the NHS, should be welcomed, since such data will not only provide us with evidence that NHS organisational culture is truly embracing a system view of failure, it should also provide us with more statistical information about the actual numbers of patients who experience unintended harm. Such information would provide greater clarity about the numbers of failures occurring across secondary, tertiary, primary and independent care. It remains to be seen however, whether a voluntary, confidential reporting system will ever really be able to provide us with a definitive picture of the numbers of patient safety failures occurring across the whole of the UK's health service industry.

References

Arah OA, Klazinga NS (2004) How safe is the safety paradigm? *Health and Safety in Health Care* **13**: 226-232

Blendon R (2002) Views of practising physicians and the public on medical error. *N Engl J Med* **347**: 1933-1940

Brennan RA, Leape LL, Laid NM et al (1991) Incidence of adverse events and negligence in hospitalised patients. Results of the Harvard Medical Practice Study

1. *N Engl J Med* **324**: 370-376

Busse DK, Wright DJ (2000) Classification and analysis of incidents in complex medical environments. *Topics in Health Information Management* **20**(4): 1-11

Carroll JS, Rudolph JW, Hatakenaka S (2002) Lessons learned from non-medical industries: root cause analysis as culture change at a chemical plant. *Quality in Health Care* **11**: 266-269

Coles J, Pryce D, Shaw C (2001) *The Reporting of Adverse Clinical Incidents — Achieving High Quality Reporting: The results of a short research study.* National Patient Safety Research Programme, University of Birmingham

De Rosier J, Stalhandske E, Bagian JP, Nudell T (2002) Using health care failure mode and effects analysis: The VA National Center for Patient Safety's Prospective Risk Analysis Scheme. *The Joint Commission Journal of Quality Improvement* **10**: 248-257

Dean B, Schachter M, Vincent C, Barber N (2002) Prescribing errors in hospital inpatients: their incidence and clinical significance. *QSHC* **11**: 340-344

DH (1997) *The New NHS: Modern, Dependable.* Stationery Office, London

DH (1998) *A First Class Service: Quality in the NHS.* Stationery Office, London

DH (2000) *An Organisation with a Memory.* Stationery Office, London

DH (2001a) *The Removal, Retention and Use of Human Organs and Tissue from Post Mortem Examinations.* Stationery Office, London

DH (2001b) *Building a Safer NHS for Patients.* Stationery Office, London

DH (2004) *Building a Safer NHS for Patients: Improving medication safety.* Stationery Office, London

Department of Health Social Services and Public Safety (2001) *Best Practice Best Care Northern Ireland.* DHSSPS, Belfast

Donchin Y, Gopher D (2003) A look into the nature and causes of human errors in the intensive care unit. *Quality and Safety in Health Care* **12**(2): 143-147

Ebright PR, Patterson ES, Render MC (2002) The 'new look' approach to patient safety: A guide for clinical nurse specialist leadership. *Clin Nurse Specialist* **16**(5): 247-253

Ek A, Olsson U, Akselsson KR (2000) *Safety Culture Onboard Ships.* Proceedings of the Human Factors and Ergonomics Society Annual Meeting, London

Evans C (2004) Anonymity and transparency in reporting of medical error: a community-based survey in South Australia. *Med J Aust* **180**: 577-580

Firth-Cozens J, Redfern N, Moss F (2001) *Confronting Errors in Patient Care: Report on Focus Groups.* National Patient Safety Research Programme, University of Birmingham

Flin R, Yule S (2003) Advances in patient safety: non-technical skills in surgery. *Surgeon News* **4**(3): 83-86

Gadd S, Colllins AM (2002) *Safety Culture: A review of the literature.* HSL/2002/25. Health and Safety Laboratory. Stationery Office, London

Gallagher T, Waterman A, Ebers A et al (2003) Patient's and physician's attitudes regarding the disclosure of medical errors. *J Am Med Assoc* **289**: 1001-1007

Gladstone J (1995) Drug administration errors: a study into the factors underlying the occurrence and reporting of drug errors in a district general hospital. *J Adv Nurs* **22**: 628-637

Glendon AI, Litherland DK (2001) Safety climate factors, groups differences and safety behaviour in road construction. *Safety Science* **39**: 157-188

Gosbee J, Anderson T (2002) Human factors engineering design can enlighten your RCA team. *Quality and Safety in Health Care* **12**(2): 119-121

Gwande AA (2003) Risk factors for retained instruments and sponges after surgery. *N Engl J Med* **348**: 229-236

Hart E, Hazelgrove J (2001) Understanding the organisational context for adverse events in health services: the role of cultural censorship. *Quality in Health Care* **10**: 257-262

Health Foundation (2004) *Patient Safety: YouGov Survey for the Health Foundation.* http://www.health.org.uk/documents/Patient_Safety_Survey_Report.pdf

Hemman EA (2002) Creating the cultures of patient safety. *J Nurs Admin* **32**(7/8): 419-427

Henrikson K, Dayton E (2006) Organisational silence and hidden threats to patient safety. *Health Services Research* **41**(4): 1539-1554

Hofer TP, Hayward RA (2002) Are bad outcomes from questionable clinical decisions preventable medical errors: A case of case iatrogenesis. *Annals of Internal Medicine* **137**(5): E327-E334

Institute of Medicine (1999) *To Err is Human: Building a safer health system.* National Academies Press. Washington DC

Institute of Medicine(2001) *Crossing the Quality Schasm: A new health system for the 21st century.* National Academy Press, Washington DC

Kennedy I (2001) T*he Report of the Public Inquiry into Children's Heart Surgery at the Bristol Royal Infirmary 1984-1995.* Stationery Office, London

Leape L (1994) Error in medicine. *J Am Med Assoc* **272**(23): 1851-1857

Leape L (2000) Reporting of medical errors: time for a reality check. *Quality in Health Care* **9**: 143-144

Leatherman S, Donaldson L, Eisenberg J (2000) International collaboration: harnessing differences to meet common needs in improving quality of care. Editorial. *Quality in Health Care* **9**: 143-145

Maxfield DJ, McMillan GR, Patterson K, Switzler A (2005) *Silence Kills — Seven Crucial Conversations for Healthcare.* Vitalsmarts, Provo, UT

Mazor K, Simon S, Yood R et al (2004) Health Plan Members' views about disclosure of medical errors. *Annals of Internal Medicine* **140**(6): 409-418

Merle V, Van Rossem V, Tayolacci MP et al (2005) Knowledge and opinions of surgical patients regarding nosocomial infections. *J Hosp Infection* **60**: 1609-1617

Meurier CE, Vincent CA, Parmar DG (1997) Learning from errors in nursing practice. *J Adv Nurs* **26**: 111-119

Millenson ML (2002) Pushing the profession: how the news media turned patient safety into a priority. *Quality Safety in Health Care* **11**: 57-63

Millenson ML (2003) The Silence. *Health Affairs* **22**(2): 103-113

Ministry of Justice (2007) *Justice for Corporate Deaths: Royal Assent for Corporate Manslaughter and Corporate Homicide Act* https://www.justice.gov.uk/news/ newsrelease260707b.htm (accessed 10 October 2007)

Mohr JJ, Batalden P, Barch P (2004) Integrating patient safety into the clinical microsystem. *Quality and Safety in Health Care* **2**: ii34-ii38

NPSA (2003) *Seven Steps to Safety: A guide for NHS staff.* NPSA, London

NPSA (2004) *Response to Health Foundation and YouGov Patient Safety Poll.* http://81.144.177.110/web/display?contentId=3333

NPSA (2005) *Building a Memory: Preventing harm, reducing risk and improving patient safety. The first report of the NRLS and the Patient Safety Observatory.* NPSA, London

National Patient Safety Foundation (1997) *Public Opinion of Patient Safety Issues: research findings.* American Medical Association, washington DC

Nolan T (2000) System changes to improve patient safety. *BMJ* **320**: 771-773

Osborne J, Blais K, Hayes JS (1999) Nurses' perceptions: When is it a medication error? *J Nurs Admin* **29**(4): 33-38

Ottewill M (2003) The current approach to human error and blame in the NHS. *Br J Nurs* **12**(15): 919-924

Reason J (1997) *Managing the Risks of Organisational Accidents.* Ashgate, Aldershot

Reason J (2000) Human error: models and management. *BMJ* **320**: 768-770

Reason J, Carthey J, de Leval MR (2001) Diagnosing 'vulnerable system syndrome': an essential pre-requisite to effective risk management. *Quality in Health Care* **10** (Supple II): ii21-ii25

Regulation Quality Improvement Authority (2006) *Project Plan for the Programme of Clinical and Social Governance Reviews: 2006-2007.* DHSSPS, Belfast

Ritchie Report (2000) *An Inquiry into Quality and Practice in the NHS Arising from the Actions of Rodney Ledward.* Stationery Office, London

Runciman W (2002) Lessons from the Australian Patient Safety Foundation: Setting up a national patient safety surveillance system: Is this the right model? *Quality and Safety in Health Care* **11**: 246-251

Runciman WB, Merryman A (2003) A tragic death: a time to blame or a time to learn? *Quality and Safety in Health Care* **112**: 321-322

Scottish Executive (2005a) *Delivering for Health.* November. B44012 11/05. Scottish Executive Health Department, Edinburgh

Scottish Executive (2005b) *Building a Health Service Fit for the Future.* May. B40206 05/05. Scottish Executive Health Department, Edinburgh

Shipman Report (2004) *Safeguarding Patients: Lessons from the past — proposals for the future. Command Paper. CM 6394*. Stationery Office, London

SHOT (2004) *Serious Hazards of Transfusion Annual Report*. www.shotuk.org/index.htm

Spink A (1004) *Patient Safety, Clinical Risk and Medical Error*. Lecture. *New Developments in Health Care Law*. Seminar. Old Hall, Lincoln's Inns, London, and European Law Research Centre, University of Salford

Vincent C, Neale G, Woloshynowych M (2001) Adverse events in British hospitals: preliminary retrospective chart review. *BMJ* **322**: 517-519

Vincent C, Taylor-Adams S, Stanhope N (1998) Framework for analysing risk and safety in clinical medicine. *BMJ* **316**: 1154-1157

Weinberg J (2002) Medical error and patient safety: understanding cultures in conflict. *Law and Policy* **24**(2): 93-113

Wilson M, Murray AE, Black MA, McDowell DA (1997) The implementation of hazard analysis and critical control points in hospital catering. *Managing Service Quality* **7**(3): 150-156

Yule S, Flin R, Paterson-Browne S, Maran N (2006) Non-technical skills for surgeons in the operating room: a review of the literature. *Surgery* **139**(2): 140-149

CHAPTER 2

Creating and Sustaining a Culture of Safety

Lynne Currie

'...many attempts to describe the nature of...culture...seem to have the definitional precision of a cloud'

James Reason, 1997

This chapter provides an overview of the importance attached to engendering a safety culture across the NHS as a way of improving the safety of patient care. It describes in some detail the differences between organisational and safety climate and culture drawing on the wider safety science literature. The chapter concludes with a consideration of some of the tools currently available to assist NHS organisations in assessing both safety culture and climate, and describes the potential benefits in utilising a safety climate assessment tool that has been developed in the UK petrochemical industry for use in NHS organisations.

Transforming NHS Culture

Following the major public inquiry into events at the Royal Bristol Infirmary (Kennedy, 2001) and the publication of *An Organisation with a Memory* (DH, 2000) much greater attention is now being paid to improving the safety of patient care across the NHS. The UK Government has formulated policy and created a national agency for patient safety, actions which are predominantly based on an understanding that patient safety failures occur as a result of poorly designed systems. The differences between taking a systemic or a traditional view of error have been described in chapter 1. The whole tone of current policies on modernising the NHS is underpinned by the concept of cultural transformation, and the requirement to focus activities away from blaming individuals when things go wrong (DH, 2000; DH. 2001). One of the most influential commentators in the patient safety movement is James Reason who has suggested there are five key attributes of a safety culture — see *Figure 2.1*.

Given the fundamental importance attached to the idea of a cultural transformation of the NHS as a way of embedding improvements in patient

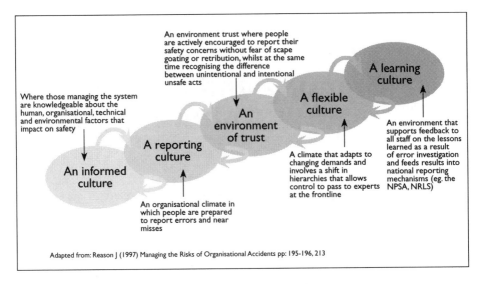

Adapted from: Reason J (1997) Managing the Risks of Organisational Accidents pp: 195-196, 213

Figure 2.1. Reason's (1997) five attributes of safety culture.

safety, there is a great need to clearly identify and articulate what is meant by an 'informed', 'reporting', 'just', 'flexible' and 'learning' culture — see *Figure 2.1*.

Whilst it is crucial to recognise the importance of taking a system approach to failure, as well as realising healthcare can never be totally error-free, it also becomes fundamentally important to acknowledge what kinds of failures should be construed as blameworthy (Bagian, 2005). It behoves us to be clear about where accountability lies within a just culture. Reason (1997) is quite clear in his articulation that while a taking a system approach to safety focuses both situational factors and latent conditions, individual accountability inevitably still has a place. In a 'just culture' individuals will still be accountable:

> *'...even though the intent is to create an atmosphere where individuals feel safe to openly report and learn from....mistakes'*
>
> Henrikson and Dayton, 2006: 1543

However, there must also be a realisation that there may well be circumstances in which blame is warranted, and if an individual's actions are proven to be negligent or unsafe, then there needs to be flexibility within the system to ensure that such individuals are dealt with appropriately. Taking a holistic system approach to failure, it may be useful to identify when and where system failures are themselves blameworthy. This brings us back to Nolan's typology (Nolan, 2000) discussed in chapter 1 around the decisions that are made, or not made, at the blunt end of care. In the case of serious safety failures, which may have been identified as being systemic in origin it may still be appropriate to invoke punitive, legal action. This type of action could be similar to that being sought in other industries, for example the attempts to charge senior managers with corporate manslaughter following the Paddington train disaster in 1999. Sometimes it is not enough to simply say that a system approach (as if the system is this amorphous thing that is just there) is being taken in the investigation of failure — almost as if this negates any further course of action.

Much has been written about the need to transform NHS culture to ensure that those working in healthcare can do so in an environment that is transparent, safe and just (DH, 1997; DH, 1998; Donaldson, 2001). Some commentators have argued that a safety culture is emerging where professionals feel able to report their concerns about poor practice and adverse events, and challenge what they perceive to be poor decisions (Ebright et al, 2002; Hemman, 2002; Bhatia et al, 2003). What is noticeable is a change of language with regard to culture, perhaps reflecting a need for a more gradual shift in thinking, and instead of advocating a no-blame culture commentators now talk about the need to inculcate a culture of fair blame, or using Reason's terminology a 'just' culture (Runciman and Merryman, 2003).

However, some commentators have suggested that embracing a 'just' culture is some way from fruition in many healthcare organisations (Weinberg, 2002; Hall, 2001). This latter view is supported by recent research undertaken both in the USA (Maxfield, et al, 2005), and the UK (Currie et al, 2007).

But exactly how do we engender a safety culture across the NHS? In order to understand more about how organisations might create and sustain a safety culture we first need to understand the trajectory and development of safety climate and safety culture, how such concepts might be investigated or assessed, as well as figuring out how these fit into concepts of organisational culture and organisational climate. In order to do this it becomes necessary to consider a wider perspective of safety science, one which has emerged from industries as diverse as petrochemicals, nuclear energy, aviation and manufacturing. However, first we must try and answer the question: what is culture?

What is Culture?

In some ways attempting to answer this question is like wading through treacle, or we can appropriate Reason's view that:

> *'...the many attempts to describe the nature of...culture must seem to have the definitional precision of a cloud'*
>
> Reason, 1997: 192

Despite the significance that policy-makers have given to culture and the cultural transformation of the NHS, they have made no meaningful attempt to define what they mean by the concept in any particular context. Policymakers unreflective, uncritical use of culture stands in marked contrast to its use within the social sciences, where defining culture has long been identified as a complex and difficult task (Savage, 2000). Although no overall consensus exists about how culture should be defined, recent thinking has shifted from one-dimensional definitions such as 'the way things are done around here', towards definitions that are far more tentative, open-ended and contentious.

In traditional accounts, the consensual, integrative, relatively static aspects of culture were emphasised, and stress was placed on shared norms, values, practices and rituals. However, recent accounts emphasise culture as the product of political processes involving the struggle of individuals or groups with unequal access to power to impose their own meaning on the world around them (Wright, 1998). As a result culture is always under construction and the processes of cultural transformation can be hampered by conflict and competition.

Organisational Culture

Organisational culture is viewed as the beliefs that an organisation's members share about the organisation, the people, and the environment in which they work (Guldenmund, 2000), or the evolution of social systems over time (Dennison, 1996). It is seen as the invisible force behind the tangibles and observables within an organisation (Ruchin et al, 2004). Culture is to an organisation what personality is to the individual; it is a hidden, yet at the same time, unifying theme that provides meaning, motivation and direction. In general terms culture is said to have three core elements:

- Basic assumptions which lie at the deepest level
- Espoused values which lie at the intermediate level
- Artefacts which lie at the surface level (Schein, 2004).

According to Guldenmund (2000) originally the term used was 'organisational climate', which referred:

'...to a global, integrating concept underlying most organisational events and processes. Nowadays, this concept is referred to by the term organisational culture whereas organisational climate has come to mean more and more the overt manifestation of culture within an organisation. Therefore, climate follows naturally from culture or, put another way organisational culture expresses itself through organisational climate'

Guldenmund, 2000: 221

Organisational Climate

'Organisational climate' has been defined as the shared characteristics of behaviour and expressed feelings of organisational members' (Guldenmund, 2000), or as the impact that organisational systems have on organisational

members' attitudes, perceptions and behaviour (Dennison, 1996, Cooper, 2000). Organisation climate is a multi-dimensional construct encompassing a range of individual evaluations of their working environment. Such evaluations may refer to general dimensions of leadership, roles and communication, or to specific dimensions like the climate for safety.

A focus on organisation climate is concerned with peoples' attitudes towards and perceptions of the organisation, whilst the focus of organisation culture is concerned with understanding the underlying structure of the symbols, myths and rituals manifested in the shared values, norms and meanings of organisational groups (Mearns and Flin, 1999). Although on the surface there appears to be clear distinctions between culture and climate, an earlier analysis of the research on organisation culture and climate suggests these distinctions become less clear, leading to the possibility that the difference may be one of interpretation, rather than one of phenomenon (Dennison, 1996).

Safety Culture

The term '*safety culture*' was first introduced by the International Atomic Energy Agency following the disaster at Chernobyl in the mid 1980s (Gadd and Collins, 2002), and arose from the detailed analyses of public enquiries following major disasters (Clark, 2000). These analyses suggested that organisations could reduce their accident rates by developing a 'positive safety culture', a term widely recognised by safety researchers (University of Loughborough, 2000; Farrington-Darby et al, 2005). Organisations with a positive safety culture are characterised by communications based on mutual trust, by shared perceptions of the importance of safety and by confidence in the efficacy of preventive measures (Ek et al, 2000; Harvey et al, 2001; Ebright et al, 2002; Hemman, 2002). In health care this notion of trust is seen as fundamental if healthcare organisations are to move towards a culture that supports the workforce in redesigning the system in order to improve both the safety and the quality of healthcare services (Berwick, 2003).

Safety culture is defined as the characteristics and attitudes in organisations and individuals which establish whether or not safety issues are given the attention justified by their significance (Guldenmund, 2000). A more global definition views it as the enduring value and priority that is placed safety by everyone working in an organisation. It refers to the extent to which individuals and groups will commit to a personal responsibility for safety, will act to preserve, enhance and communicate any safety concerns, will strive to learn, adapt and modify — both individual and organisational — behaviour based on the lessons that are learned from failure, and be rewarded in a manner consistent with those values (Weigman et al, 2002).

However, safety culture may also be viewed differently by different groups working in an organisation. For example, in a hospital healthcare professionals may hold different views about the culture of the organisation to those of managers. These different groups may in fact view safety through their own sub-culture, and as such there may be no shared overall view of safety (Ebright et al, 2002). Subcultures however, can also be positive because they offer different perspectives and diversity, which can lead to the effective communication of risk (Mearns et al, 1997). Sub-cultures may prove to be valuable in dealing with collective ignorance because they may also provide different interpretations of emerging safety problems (Cooper, 2000). However, the reality of professional sub-cultures, each with potentially differing views about what constitutes improvements in safety, may prove challenging when attempting to transform the culture in healthcare organisations.

Safety Climate

The term '*safety climate*' was first introduced in 1980 (Cooper and Phillips, 2004), and is defined as shared employee perceptions of how safety management is being operationalised in the workplace at a particular moment in time. Safety climate is characterised as being temporal and state-like, making it more open to assessment and change (Cheyne et al, 1998). Climate has been referred to as workers' attitudes towards safety (Mearns et al, 1999; Rundmo, 2001; Cheyne et al, 2002) and has been identified as a useful indicator of the way safety is managed across an organisation (Cox and Flin, 1998). A more global definition defines safety climate as the temporal measure of safety culture which is situationally based and refers to the perceived state of safety at a particular place at a particular time. As such safety climate is relatively unstable and is subject to change depending on the current environment and prevailing conditions (Weigman et al, 2002). Therefore, assessing a hospital's safety climate is a bit like taking its safety temperature (Glendon and Litherland, 2001).

Given the complexity and multi-dimensionality of the concepts of safety culture and safety climate, *Figure 2.2* outlines the relations that may affect staffs' perceptions of safety climate, their understanding of the safety culture within their organisation, and ultimately their individual safety behaviour.

Understanding the Role of Culture in Patient Safety

The safety science literature is replete with definitions and terminologies related to the concepts of safety climate and safety culture, with many commentators arguing that the fragmented and unsystematic nature safety research is due to the lack of an underlying integrative framework (Pidgeon, 1997, 1998; Cooper, 2000; Neal et al, 2000; Clarke, 2000; Guldenmund, 2000; Hale, 2000).

Pidgeon (1997, 1998) argues that during the 1970s Turner explicated a theory of man-made disasters observing that organisations function in relation

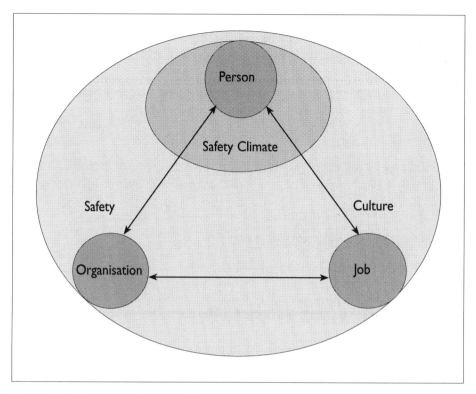

Figure 2.2. Relations affecting staff perceptions of safety climate in healthcare organisations.

to a range of cultural beliefs and norms about safety and safety management, some of which can be made explicit through formal policies and procedures, and some of which can be more tacitly understood and entrenched within everyday working practices. However, over time there may be a incubation period where latent errors — which are at odds with the prevailing cultural assumptions about safety — combine over time to make organisations vulnerable to catastrophe. Any catastrophe that befalls an organisation is then seen as an acknowledgment that the existing cultural beliefs held about safety have become dislodged or have broken down (Pidgeon, 1997).

Turner's allusion to culture in his theory of man-made disasters was, according to Pidgeon (1997), 15 years ahead of its time and predates many of the current discussions and theories circulating about risk and culture in NHS organisations, and it provides the conceptual foundation for a definition of safety culture (Pidgeon, 1997). Turner believed that while it may be convenient to talk about cultures of safety on a continuum from 'good' to 'bad' the unacknowledged paradox inherent within culture is that is can act both as a precondition for safe and unsafe operations. What this means is that the culture within an organisation can seriously impact on the way safety is, or is not effectively managed. This is the case because patient safety failures do not happen by chance, they arise over time as a result of relations between:

> '...the human and organisational arrangements of the socio-technical systems set up to manage complex and ill-structured risk problems...'
>
> Pidgeon, 1997: 205

While this type of argument may have been viewed as strange in the late 1970s, it has greatly contributed to how contemporary analysts now view patient safety failures as being:

> '...managerial and administrative in origin'
>
> Pidgeon, 1997: 205

Methods of Assessing Safety Culture

Given the complexity and diversity in the relationship between safety climate and safety culture, it is possible to see that these two concepts are distinct yet closely related. Such distinctions presuppose a need to differentiate between approaches and methods that can be utilised to assess safety culture and safety climate.

Clarke (2000) has identified four approaches to measuring culture which include attitudinal based interventions; behaviour modification; implementation of a safety culture; and implementation of total safety management.

Attitudinal-based interventions can be carried out using a baseline measurement of safety climate, whereby the baseline measurement is followed up with a programme of patient safety improvement interventions, followed by a second measurement of safety climate. What organisations would be looking for between the first and second measurement is evidence of move towards a more positive attitude to safety (Clarke, 2000).

Behaviour modification is underpinned by a need to identify a range of critical safety behaviours, and such behaviours can be identified through the use of in-depth interviews and observations of practice in addition to setting targets for improvements and providing regular feedback on performance. What organisations would be looking for from a programme of behaviour modification would be a reduction in unsafe behaviours, leading again to more positive attitudes towards safety (Clarke, 2000).

Implementing a total safety management culture whereby behavioural changes happen only occurs when employees are actively involved in safety, and it requires a clear identification of those people who are most likely to change their behaviour (Clarke, 2000). Taking forward a programme of total safety management as a way of transforming culture requires a more sustained focus on the underlying cause of accidents which will bring greater benefits to the organisation (Clarke, 2000).

Understanding the Role of Climate in Patient Safety

The safety climate of an organisation has been identified as useful for predicting safety-related outcomes like accidents and incidents (Glendon and Litherland, 2001). Some of the major disasters that have taken place in other industries have led researchers to focus on the importance of work climates and management practices which are increasingly being seen as determinants of safety in the workplace (Neal and Griffiths, 2006).

The ability to predict accidents and incidents is important, because until recently many organisations have used what have been identified as 'lagging indicators' (also referred to as trailing indicators) to explore organisational safety (Flin et al, 2000). Lagging indicators rely on retrospective data and are identified as counting the number of fatalities, accident rates and near misses (Flin et al, 2000).

In non-health industries there has been a move away from safety measures based on retrospective data or 'lagging indicators' such as fatalities, accident rates and incidents, to a more predictive model of exploring organisational safety which turns on the idea of looking at 'leading indicators', (sometimes referred to as safety metrics). Such leading indicators are identified as measurements of safety climate or safety audits (Flin et al, 2000). Using these types of predictive measures enables safety condition monitoring without having to wait for the system to fail before applying remedial action, and they are predicated on a switch from 'feedback' to 'feedforward' controls (Flin et al, 2000).

In health care the preoccupation with safety has only recently become more focused as a result of the global importance now placed on patient safety. As such, it can be argued that endeavours to improve patient safety in the NHS lean towards the reporting of lagging indicators, reflected in efforts to report clinical incidents, adverse events, and near misses. This is evidenced by the rollout of the National Patient Safety Agency's (NPSA) National Reporting and Learning System (NRLS) and the emphasis being placed on root cause analysis which has been described in chapter 1.

While the NHS doubtless has some catching up to do in relation to the measures being propagated across the nuclear, petrochemical and manufacturing industries, recent thinking by James Reason has focused on the importance of 'error wisdom' and the transferability of what he calls 'mental skills' (Reason, 2004). He argues that although frontline clinical staff are provided with little

'...opportunity to make radical changes to the system [we could] ...provide them with some basic mental skills that would help them to recognise and if possible, avoid situations with a high error potential'

Reason, 2004: 31

This work has been taken forward by the National Patient Safety Agenda in its development of a Foresight Training Programme (NPSA, 2006)

Methods of Assessing Safety Climate

In assessing safety climate organisations could measure workers attitudes and perceptions of safety across a range of factors, including management and supervision, the safety system, risk, work pressures, and competencies (Cooper, 2000). There are a number of safety climate questionnaires that have been developed for use across different industries including road construction, (Glendon and Litherland, 2001) manufacturing, (Cheyne et al, 2002; Cooper, 2004), petrochemical/oil (Cheyne et al, 1998; Cox and Cheyne, 2000; University of Loughborough Business School, 2000), and steel (Prussia et al, 2000), and one of these, the Safety Climate Questionnaire (SCQ), has been tested for use in an NHS setting (Currie et al, 2007).

The early safety climate assessment tools measured staffs attitudes and perceptions across six factors (Zohar, 1980; Glendon and Litherland, 2001) but more recent instruments have used between nine and two factors (Cox and Cheyne, 2000; Rundmo, 2000). Debate continues about whether it is possible to identify a universal or generic set of stable safety climate factors that could apply across all organisations and industries. Coyle et al (1995) argue that while no universal set of safety climate factors exist, others disagree, suggesting that:

'...some safety climate factors...might be stable across both industries and cultures'

Glendon and Litherland, 2001: 174

A number of common factors have emerged from various studies, and these are identified as management/supervision; safety system, risk, work pressure, and competence (Clarke, 2000; Mearns et al, 2001).

Questionnaires are useful tools in the measurement of safety climate because they provide a snapshot of the organisation's state of safety as discerned through the attitudes and perceptions of the workforce at a particular moment in time (Mearns, et al, 1997). This provides a way of seeing changes in the atmosphere of the workplace and gives an indication of the way safety is managed (Cox and Flin, 1998).

The Safety Climate Questionnaire (SCQ)

The Safety Climate Questionnaire is an element of the Safety Climate Measurement User Guide and Toolkit developed for use in the UK petrochemical industry. The Toolkit is based on a systems approach to organisational culture, and it is a multi-method package to help researchers investigate culture from a more holistic perspective incorporating elements of organisational structure, function and behaviour (Cox and Cheyne, 2000). The full Toolkit includes questionnaires, focus groups, behavioural observations and situational audits to describe and explore the efficacy of health and safety management systems (Cox and Cheyne, 2000), and it is downloadable at www.lboro.ac.uk/departments/bs/safety/documents.pdf.

The process of developing the original SCQ was undertaken by researchers working at the Centre for Hazard and Risk Management at the University of Loughborough's Business School, and a detailed description of this process, can be found in Cox and Cheyne (2000).

The SCQ was tested for use in an NHS setting in a large purpose-built teaching NHS hospital in the UK (Currie et al, 2007). The SCQ consists of 43 items and measures staffs' attitudes to safety climate using nine dimensions, which include:

- Management commitment
- Communication
- Priority of safety
- Safety rules and procedures
- Supportive environment
- Involvement
- Personal priorities and need for safety
- Personal appreciation of risk
- Work environment.

Currie et al's (2007) findings indicate that the SCQ has proved to be a highly reliable instrument for measuring safety climate across a large complex NHS hospital. Whilst the consistency of the dimensions measured by safety climate questionnaires may be context or organisation specific, if the SCQ was utilised across a range of similar NHS organisations it would be possible to accumulate a core database of organisational safety climate profiles, which could be used to benchmark best practice. Benchmarking safety climate would not only help organisations to identify areas for improvements in safety, it would provide motivation for staff who are involved in managing risk, and assist organisations in managing patient safety more effectively.

References

Bagian JP (2005) Patient safety: what is really at issue? *Frontiers Health Services Management* **22**(1): 3-16

Berwick DM (2003) Improvement, trust and the healthcare workforce. *Quality and Safety in Health Care* **12**: 448-452

Bhatia R, Blackshaw G et al (2003) Developing a departmental culture for reporting adverse events. *International Journal of Health Care Quality* **16**(3): 154-156

Cheyne A, Cox S, Oliver A, Tomas JM (1998) Modelling safety climate in the prediction of levels of safety activity. *Work and Stress* **12**(3): 255-271

Cheyne A, Oliver A, Tomas JM, Cox S (2002) The architecture of employee attitudes to safety in the manufacturing sector. *Personnel Review* **31**(5/6): 649-669

Clarke S (2000) Safety culture: under-specified and overrated? *International Journal of Management Review* **2**(1): 65-90

Cooper D (2000) Towards a model of safety culture. *Safety Science* **36**: 111-136

Cooper MD, Phillips RA (2004) Exploratory analysis of the safety climate and safety behaviour relationship. *Journal of Safety Research* **35**: 497-512

Cox S, Cheyne AJT (2000) Assessing safety culture in offshore environments. *Safety Science* **34**(1-3): 111–129

Cox S J, Flin R (1998) Safety culture: Philosopher's stone or man of straw? *Work and Stress* **2**(3): 189-201

Coyle IR, Sleeman SD, Admas N (1995) Safety climate. *J Safety Research* **26**: 247–54

Currie VL, Cooper C, Watterson L (2007) *A Survey of Staffs' Attitudes to Safety Climate*. RCN Institute, Oxford

Dennison DR (1996) What is the difference between organisational culture and organisational climate? A native's point of view on a decade of paradigm wars. *Academy of Management Review* **31**(3): 619-654

DH (1997) *The New NHS: Modern, Dependable*. Stationery Office, London

DH (1998) *A First Class Service: Quality in the NHS*. Stationery Office, London

DH (2000) *An Organisation with a Memory*. Stationery Office, London

DH (2001) *Building a Safer NHS*. Stationery Office, London

Donaldson LJ (2001) Clinical governance: a mission to improve. *Clinical Performance and Quality Health Care* **8**(1): 6-8

Ebright PR, Patterson ES et al (2002) The 'new look' approach to patient safety: a guide for clinical nurse specialist leadership. *Clin Nurse Specialist* **16**(5): 247-253

Ek A, ,Olsson U, Akselsson KR (2000) *Safety Culture Onboard Ships*. Proceedings of the Human Factors and Ergonomics Society Annual Meeting, London

Farrington-Darby T, Pickup L, Wilson JR (2005) Safety culture in railway maintenance. *Safety Science* **43**: 39-60

Flin R, Mearns K, O'Connor P, Bryden R (2000) Measuring safety climate:

Identifying the common features. *Safety Science* **34**: 177-193

Gadd S, Collins AM (2002) *Safety Culture: A review of the literature.* Health and Safety Laboratory https://www.hse.gov.uk/research/hs/02.25.pdf (accessed 15 December 2006)

Glendon AI, Litherland DK (2001) Safety climate factors, groups differences and safety behaviour in road construction. *Safety Science* **39**: 157-188

Guldenmund FW (2000) The nature of safety culture: A review of theory and research. *Safety Science* **34**: 215-257

Hale AR (2000) Culture's Confusions. *Safety Science* **34**: 1-14

Hall D (2001) No blame should be apportioned in corporate failure. *BMJ* **323**: 732

Harvey J, Bolam H, Gregory D, Erdos G (2001) The effectiveness of training to change safety culture within a highly regulated environment. *Personnel Review* **30**(6): 615-636

Hemman EA (2002) Creating the cultures of patient safety. *J Nurs Admin* **32**(7/8): 419-427

Henrikson K, Dayton E (2006) Organisational silence and hidden threats to patient safety. *Health Services Research* **41**(4): Part II: 1539-1554

Kennedy I (2001) *Learning from Bristol: The Report of the Public Inquiry into Children's Heart Surgery at the Bristol Royal Infirmary 1984-1995.* Stationery Office, London

Maxfield DJ, McMillan GR, Patterson K, Switzler A (2005) *Silence Kills — Seven Crucial Conversations for Healthcare.* Vitalsmarts, Provo, UT

Mearns K, Flin R, Fleming M, Gordon R (1997) *Organisational and Human Factors in Offshore Safety.* Health and Safety Executive, London

Mearns KJ, Flin R (1999) Assessing the state of organisational safety — culture or climate? *Current Psychology* **18**(1): 5-17

Mearns K Flin R, O'Connor P (2001) Sharing 'worlds at risk': improving communication with crew resource management. *Journal of Risk Research* **4**(4): 377-392

Meek VL (1988) Organisational culture: origins and weaknesses. *Organisational Studies* **9**(4): 453-473

NPSA (2006) *Learn from the Past, but Look to the Future: Strategies for Improving Foresight.* http://www.saferhealthcare.org.uk/IHI/Topics/ManagingChange/Features/4481_LearningFromThePast.htm (accessed 1 March 2007).

Neal A, Griffin MA, Hart PM (2000) The impact of organisational climate on safety climate and individual behaviour. *Safety Science* **34**: 99-109

Neal A, Griffin MA (2006) A study of the lagged relationships among safety climate, safety motivation, safety behaviour, and accidents at the individual level and group levels. *J Applied Psychol* **91**(4): 946-953

Nolan T (2000) System changes to improve patient safety. *BMJ* **320**: 771–3

Pidgeon N (1997) The limits to safety? Culture, politics, learning and man-made disasters. *J Contingencies and Crisis Management* **5**(1): 1-14

Pidgeon N (1998) Safety culture: key theoretical issues. *Work and Stress* **12**(3): 202-216

Prussia GE, Brown KA, Willis PG (2003) Mental models of safety: do managers and employees see eye to eye? *J Safety Research* **34**: 143-156

Axtell-Ray CA (1986) Corporate culture: the last frontier of control? *J Management Studies* **23**(3): 287-297

Reason J (1997) *Managing the Risks of Organisational Accidents.* Ashgate, Aldershot

Reason J (2004) Beyond the organisational accident: the need for 'error wisdom' on the frontline. *Quality and Safety in Health Care* **13**: 28-33

Rundmo T (2000) Safety climate: attitudes and risk perception in Norsk Hydro. *Safety Science* **34**: 47-59

Ruchlin HS (2004) The role of leadership is instilling a culture of safety: lessons from the literature. *J Healthcare Management* **49**(1): 47-58

Runciman WB, Merryman A (2003) A tragic death: a time to blame or a time to learn? *Quality and Safety in Health Care* **112**: 321-322

Savage J (2000) The culture of 'culture' in National Health Service policy implementation. *Nursing Inquiry* **7**: 230-238

Schein E (2004) *Organisational Culture and Leadership.* 3rd edn. Jossey-Bass. San Francisco

University of Loughborough (2000) *Safety Climate Measurement User Guide and Toolkit.* www.lboro.ac.uk/departments/bs/safety.documents.pdf (accessed 29 November 2006)

Wiegmann DA, Zhang H, von Thaden T, Sharma G, Mitchell A (2002) *A Synthesis of Safety Culture and Safety Climate Research.* Institute of Aviation Technical Report, University of Illinois http://www.humanfactors.uiuc.edu/ Reports&PapersPDFs/TechReport/02-3.pdf (accessed 28th November, 2006)

Weinberg J (2002) Medical error and patient safety: understanding cultures in conflict. *Law and Policy* **24**(2): 93-113

Wright S (1998) Politicisation of 'culture'. *Anthropology in Action* **5**(1/2): 3-10

Zohar D (1980) Safety climate in industrial organisations: theoretical and applied applications. *J Applied Psychol* **65**(1): 96-102

Professions, Organisations and Patient Safety: Stories of Malicious and Inept Practice

Frank Milligan

What constitutes a profession and a professional are questions that ignite intense interest in some practitioners, but will leave many others wondering when they can get back to doing some real work. Yet, they are questions that are relevant to patient safety. As the case of the late General Practitioner (GP) Harold Shipman has shown, there are some vitally important edges to this debate that impact upon patient safety. As described in chapter 1, the challenge of achieving significant improvements in patient safety is one of the key tasks facing healthcare at the start of the 21st century. There is broad international agreement on the nature of the task faced and the importance of achieving improvements to quality in this area (Kohn et al, 2000; DH, 2001; DH, 2004; National Health Performance Committee, 2004). The estimated 25,000 preventable deaths from adverse events in the National Health Service (NHS) each year (Bristol Royal Infirmary Inquiry, 2001) is testimony to the notion that things are not what they should be and perhaps professions, so called professionals and the organisations within which they work are not, to put it crudely, doing a good job.

This chapter will not dwell for too long on sociological debates on professions and the ramifications of professional status. It will however explore the professional, and to a lesser extent the organisational and bureaucratic, patient safety inadequacies that tragic cases described here have highlighted. These cases are used here as another means through which the suffering of the patients involved, and that of their families and friends, can be acknowledged and used in a positive way for learning. Although the case studies illustrated here are medical staff, they hold lessons for all healthcare practitioners, especially nurses who have historically worked so closely with doctors. One of the more controversial points that will be made is that we cannot rely on professional status to improve patient safety; indeed, it is often a significant barrier that advantages the profession and its members as opposed to the patient.

The aim of this chapter is to explore the role of so called professions and individual professionals in patient safety, especially within the context of multidisciplinary teams, organisational work and regulation. It is assumed for the purposes of this chapter that medicine is a profession and that nursing is still striving for professional status. It is not assumed that the latter would be a positive step forward for users of health care, whom for convenience I will refer to as patients. On this last point and for reasons of simplicity, the term patient is used to cover all users of health care.

To Do No Harm

It assumed here that the broad aim of health care is to assist people in achieving health including supporting them through the various health crises that they may face. Although such an assumption hides a number of problems, not least of which is the level of priority given to prevention as opposed to treatment, it logically leads to the conclusion that healthcare interventions should be, on balance, good for the user of health services. A balance inevitably has to be struck between the harm incurred in some of the interventions used, for example the physical harm of surgery or the side-effects of drug therapy, and the health benefits being sought. Usually the gains in the latter will outweigh the various harms and risks inherent in the care and treatment interventions used.

Sharpe and Faden (1998) in their historical analysis of medical harm give a useful examination of the oath of Hippocrates; the obligation to do no harm. They explore the balance described above and point out that the Hippocratic obligation has a very practical purpose, in that causing significant unnecessary harm would make it less likely that the patient would come back for further treatment (they might also be dead of course!). They also note that the way in which the obligation is interpreted is relative to the historical circumstances within which medical decisions are made. This is an important point as a shift was seen at the turn of the century, a shift that acknowledged patient safety as a legitimate concern of healthcare practitioners. It became clear that significant unnecessary harm, harm beyond that inevitably incurred with effective and appropriate care and treatment, was occurring along with unacceptably high error rates. The new agenda that allowed us to capture that harm is patient safety.

The Patient Safety Agenda

In the UK some of the most significant events in the emergence of the patient safety agenda were the Harold Shipman case (Baker, 2001; Smith, 2002; 2003;

2003a; 2004; 2004a; 2005), the Bristol Royal Infirmary Inquiry (2001; DH, 2002), and publication of *An Organisation with a Memory* (DH, 2000; DH, 2001). One of the recommendations from *An Organisation with a Memory*, the Chief Medical Officer's report into shortcomings in patient safety in the NHS, was the creation of a body dedicated to improving patient safety in England and Wales, the National Patient Safety Agency (NPSA). The NPSA has now established links with Northern Ireland. From an international perspective patient safety is high on the healthcare agenda (Comptroller and Auditor General, 2005), with the creation of the NPSA being seen as a significant and positive step forward, one that has yet to be achieved in some other countries (Arah and Klazinga, 2004).

Large numbers of people continue to be successfully cared for and treated by the health service in the UK, but there are a significant number of errors and other forms of unnecessary harm that occur (Milligan and Robinson, 2003; Comptroller and Auditor General, 2005). The NPSA uses the term 'patient safety incidents', although 'adverse event' has been commoner in the literature. A patient safety incident is defined as:

'Any unintended or unexpected incident which could have or did lead to harm for one or more patients receiving NHS funded care'

NPSA, 2004: 1

The NPSA included the concept of 'near miss' in its definition of a patient safety incident. These are situations that could have resulted in an accident, injury or illness for a patient but were avoided by chance or by intervention. Common patient safety incidents include, for example:

- Hospital acquired infections
- Adverse drug events (prescription errors, adverse drug reactions and drug administration errors)
- Patient falls
- Patients committing suicide and other forms of deliberate self-harm (whilst receiving healthcare interventions)
- Failure to identify and promptly treat patients who are becoming seriously ill, for example the patient who lapses into septic shock following surgery
- Intravenous fluid overload
- Giving the wrong unit of blood to a patient (mismatch).

There are many more examples, including aspects of the case studies that follow, and no doubt the reader can add their own examples. The National Audit Office (Comptroller and Auditor General, 2005) reported that an analysis of 256 NHS acute, ambulance and mental health Trusts' responses to a survey showed that some 885,832 incidents and near misses were reported in 2003-04. The follow up survey found that this had increased to around 974,000 reported incidents in 2004-05. It is important to acknowledge that an increase in reported incidents is a positive step forward in enhancing safety as the opportunity to understand and learn from them is enhanced (NPSA, 2005b). It was noted that few Trusts included hospital acquired infections in the reports and so an estimated 300,000 additional incidents probably occurred (Comptroller and Auditor General, 2005). The most common reports were in relation to patient falls, equipment, documentation and communication error. The National Audit Office estimated that the financial cost of patient safety incidents is around £2 billion a year in extra bed days with a further £1 billion incurred through hospital acquired infections. Settled clinical negligence claims cost the NHS £423 million in 2003-4. Details on the latest results from the National Reporting and Learning System, which is receiving over 50,000 patient safety incident reports a month at the time of writing (NPSA, 2006), can be found on the NPSA web site (http://www.npsa.nhs.uk/).

The Harvard Medical Practice Study (Brennan et al, 1991; Leape et al, 1991), a seminal work in patient safety, found that nearly 4% of patients suffered a patient safety incident (iatrogenic injury) that either prolonged their hospital stay or resulted in measurable injury. The Harvard Study used the concept of iatrogenic injury as opposed to patient safety incidents. Iatrogenic is defined in the Oxford English Dictionary (Second Edition 1989) as:

'Induced unintentionally by a physician through his diagnosis, manner, or treatment; of or pertaining to the induction of (mental or bodily) disorders, symptoms etc, in this way'

Oxford English Dictionary, 1989

For clarification of this concept see Sharpe and Faden (1998) and Milligan (2003) as the definition of patient safety used by the NPSA does not embrace all elements of iatrogenic injury.

Leape (1999) went on to use the calculation made in the Harvard Medical Practice Study to draw an analogy with aviation, one of the safety critical industries increasingly compared with health care. If the injury rates found in the Harvard Medical Practice Study held for the whole of the USA then 180,000 people a year would die partly as a result of patient safety incidents, the equivalent of three jumbo jet crashes every two days! Leap's point, apart from highlighting how safe in comparison aviation is, was to emphasise the high error rates and hidden nature of the problem in health care. Even though the findings of the Harvard study were quite shocking in terms of the levels of injury being caused, little obvious interest or action followed. It took another nine years before patient safety really gained momentum as evidenced by the *To err is human* report in the US (Kohn et al, 2000), and the publication of *An Organisation with a Memory* in the UK (DH, 2000).

The Harvard methods (Brennan et al, 1991; Leape et al, 1991) have been used as the basis for research into patient safety incidents in the UK (Vincent et al, 2001) and other countries, for example Australia (Wilson et al, 1995). The calculation methods used in the Harvard Study, retrospective reviews of patient records by a panel of expert practitioners, were also used by the Bristol Royal Infirmary Inquiry team in their investigation into poor survival rates in children following cardiothoracic surgery. They estimated the total possible number of annual deaths within NHS hospitals from preventable adverse events in an attempt to put the problems of the Bristol case into a national context. The Inquiry team calculated that the number of preventable deaths in the NHS would be around 25,000 a year (Bristol Royal Infirmary Inquiry, 2001).

The National Audit Office reported that around 5,000 patient deaths a year are attributable to hospital acquired infections (Comptroller and Auditor General, 2004) meaning that more people die of this preventable complication than die in road traffic accidents. The latter was calculated as 3,508 deaths in Great Britain in 2003. This was a slight rise over the previous year, but the overall trend was downwards making us one of the safer countries in Europe (Department for Transport, 2004). The opposite is true when it comes to hospital acquired infections, for example methicillin resistant *Staphylococcus aureus* (MRSA). The UK is, at the time of writing, one of the worst countries in Europe when it comes to reported *Staphylococcus aureus bacteraemias* and the incidence in 2004 was reported as being on the increase (Comptroller and Auditor General, 2004). Hospital acquired infections inevitably carry a significant cost for the NHS, at least £1 billion a year in addition to the suffering inflicted on the patient.

It can be seen from this brief review of the nature and frequency of patient safety incidents that they inevitably generate significant levels of unnecessary harm for patients yet attempts to enhance our understanding of the nature and extent of the problem are only now growing in momentum. If the aim of healthcare professions is to promote health, why has this happened?

Safety Critical Industries

The delay in seeing patient safety as a priority is in part explained by the increasing weight of evidence with regard to the size and nature of the problem and the change in perspective that has occurred in health care involving increasing comparisons with what are termed safety critical industries. The analogy given above by Leape (1999) of deaths in the USA from patient safety incidents being the equivalent of three jumbo jet crashes every two days is representative of that shift. Other fields embraced in the safety literature include the railway, nuclear power and chemical industries. It is an important step for healthcare staff to accept that although there are differences, and health care faces some unique challenges in promoting patient safety, there is much to learn from these industries (Reason, 2004). However, professions and professionals are not good at accepting and utilising the knowledge and skills of others, as they are, supposedly, experts in their own field. Yet, it is clear that those working in health care and the various professions it embraces, must learn and utilise lessons from elsewhere in the attempt to significantly improve patient safety (Leape, 1999; Reason, 2004).

The extent of the changes required in health care can be difficult to grasp for those new to the concept of patient safety, but is evident in this quotation from a book on enhancing safety culture in industry:

'What a learning environment means in practice is the existence of an ideal total work environment that strives to be safety conscious in every aspect. The whole work-related system emphasizes and pays unending attention to safety, in all aspects of design, operation, management, and rewards. Thus, the management, organizational structure, staff training, plant condition, trust, free communication, open reporting, blameless appraisal and self-criticism, awareness and readiness, and pay raises all constitute a 'culture' that reinforces and rewards safe operation'

Duffy and Saull 2003: 101

It is clear that the majority of healthcare systems across the world, and the NHS in no exception, are some way off achieving this type of learning environment although significant progress in patient safety is being made through the clinical governance agenda and the creation of the National Patient Safety Agency (NPSA). Any claims that a safety culture exists in the NHS are, on current evidence, premature.

An integral part of achieving a safety culture, as implied through the learning environment described by Duffy and Saul (2003) above, is recognition of the fact that we make errors because it is an intrinsic human trait — that to err is human (Kohn et al, 2000). An acceptance of this stance in safety critical industries such as aviation (Leape, 1999; Wiegmann and Shappell, 2003) has led to the achievement of significant improvements in safety. The focus within adverse event analysis, situations in which error and other forms of harm occur in safety critical industries, has moved from a propensity for individual blame to a systems approach. It is accepted that human, organisational, equipment and design factors can all play a part when things go wrong. This systems approach, as it is called, helps the worker to understand their own vulnerability to error and the place and influence of a range of quite diverse organisational and design issues in terms of the origins and prevention of error. This systems awareness along with an understanding that to err is human — Reason (2004) refers to the latter as 'error wisdom' — has been lacking in health care and will need to become an integral part of professional and bureaucratic regulation and process.

'Error wisdom' is evident in the *Incident Decision Tree* (go to www. npsa.nhs.uk), a tool produced by the NPSA for managers of staff involved in patient safety incidents. It guides the manager on the action, if any, to be taken against staff involved in patient safety incidents. The majority of cases analysed using the Incident Decision Tree will be found to be due to systems failures as opposed to malicious or inept practice (examples of these follow). It is important to be open and fair and not blame staff, unless they have been reckless or malicious in their actions, as this will facilitate honest and increased reporting and a subsequent reduction in patient safety incidents (Leape, 1999). The NPSA sees this as a particularly important point and launched the *Being Open* (NPSA, 2005; 2005a) initiative as a means through which to reduce the 'hiding' of incidents that has historically occurred in health care (Bristol Royal Infirmary Inquiry, 2001; DH, 2001). *Being Open* also means active patient involvement, and as will be shown, this is important in reducing the risks from malicious and inept professional practice.

The emphasis on 'error wisdom' and system explanations for errors is evident from the outset in education and training programmes in safety critical industries. Human factors theory, which includes for example types of error, lapses, the effects of stress and fatigue (Vincent and Reason, 1999), is taught from the start to new staff but this has generally not been the case in healthcare. Less constructive attitudes have been perpetuated, particularly in medicine (Sharpe and Faden, 1998), and have therefore been more generally evident in healthcare (see for example the Bristol Royal Infirmary Inquiry, 2001). Changes are now being made to the medical curriculum in the UK that embrace elements of the patient safety agenda, and it is likely that other healthcare professions will need to follow this example if they have not started to do so already.

What is a Profession and who is a Professional?

Our awareness of the patient safety agenda has developed within the context of a healthcare system made up of various professions, the most notable of which is medicine. To make sense of what professions might add to patient safety it is necessary to define what a profession might be. Robinson (2003) notes that one of the ways in which occupations (medicine was the focus of her chapter) have attempted to manage the risks involved in their practice is through demanding and securing the status of a profession. The risks referred to by Robinson were broad and related to both the users of the profession, the need to prepare practitioners who can practice in a competent manner, and the risks for the individual practitioner: that they might be subject to malicious or ill informed allegations against their character, performance or behaviour. Individuals within a profession are 'allowed' to do things that other people cannot and, importantly, they define what these things are (Hughes, 1993). Doctors and dentists, for example, do things to patient's which in another context would count as a very serious assault. Savage (1987) has made the same point in relation to nursing practice. The practitioner is not granted permission for this by the patient on the basis of an individual claim to knowledge or competence, but because of the trust generated by the practitioners membership of a profession. The patient presumes the profession owns a knowledge base that is relevant to their health and that knowledge is not accessible elsewhere (Robinson, 2003).

The safeguards put in place by a profession should, and generally do, lower risk to both public and the individual professional. These safeguards include standards of competence for initial entry to the profession, the provision of codes of practice, requirements for continuing professional development and other forms of regulation including procedures for dealing with failing members of the profession. These safeguards should solve the problem for the public of deciding who might or might not be a safe practitioner: they, the public, should be able to go to the professional confident that they will be safely and honestly supported and helped.

Membership also gives the professional a sense of identity and solidarity. The members of the profession, what Hughes (1993) refers to as the 'charmed circle', serve the public in exchange for money, goods or services. In doing this the profession will seek not just to define what is proper work for its members but what is proper conduct for the public. It is this level of influence that separates a profession from an occupation. If a profession is successful in gaining the trust of the public, which would be evident in the influence it has over the beliefs the public hold in relation to its work, its power and control over the public is enhanced as is the level of reward gained. This ability, for professions to define what is legitimate work/expertise for its members, leads back to the question posed earlier in the chapter: why has it taken so long for patient safety to be acknowledged as a priority in a healthcare system dominated by the profession of medicine?

Sociological analysis of what constitutes a profession has identified some key characteristics that are helpful to the analysis given here. The approach relies on the idea that there are certain core traits that underpin the claim to being a profession. Definitions of these traits does vary a little but they usually include the ability to:

- Control entry to the profession
- Define the portfolio of appropriate tasks to be undertaken
- Control the boundaries with other occupations
- Define the knowledge base
- Define a code of practice or ethics (Robinson, 2003).

Nursing, in comparison with medicine, has less control over some of these factors. The portfolio of tasks, for example, is frequently dictated by medicine in its delegation of work to nursing staff. The traits listed above are very much about control, inclusion and exclusion, and this has implications for other groups within society, most notably patients. It creates, to put it crudely, an 'us and them' situation; you are either a member of the professional group with the privileges and responsibilities it brings or you belong to another occupational/ professional group and/or the public.

The trait theory of professions has its critics who argue it is based on a false premise (Robinson, 2003): that the traits may well define the characteristics of existing professions, but the suggestion that the possession of these characteristics is the primary cause of the attainment of professional status fails to acknowledge other political, economic and gender imperatives (see for example Davies, 1995). The idea that professional status can be attained by simply adopting particular traits is therefore called into question. A more important issue in the context of patient safety is that in so far as nursing or any other group attains these characteristics, it may well have to discard other values.

Sharpe and Faden (1998), in their comprehensive analysis of medical harm, make it clear that medical loyalties have historically become divided between the patient and the profession, with the former often being of secondary importance to the aims of the profession. Robinson (2003) also notes that professionals can privilege the problem of their immediate client over the collective problems of the community and this may in part explain why patient safety has not, until recently, been seen as a priority by medicine. The emphasis for medicine has been on treatment of the patient rather than broader, and in some respects more everyday, yet important, organisational and design factors that might negatively impact upon patient safety. Hospital acquired infection is a practical example. A good deal of medical attention and effort has been given over to the prescription of various medications, but hospital design in this country has failed to keep up with the challenges of hospital acquired infection and other design related aspects of patient safety (Ulrich et al, 2004).

Threats to Patient Safety: The Malicious and Inept Professional

From the analysis given above it can be seen that patient safety has not, until recent times, been seen as a distinct and significant issue of concern. This is interesting in the context of professional regulation as the primary goal of any healthcare profession should be to promote health. As mentioned earlier, one of the key functions of a profession is the task of supporting and protecting its members. The support offered helps the professional meet the demands of practice and carries them through those difficult times when things might not be going well in their career. This function includes protecting the professional from malicious allegations and/or representation during investigations into their conduct or competence. This support and protection is necessary, especially as healthcare staff are inevitably involved in work that carries risks. As noted, risks include the difficult decisions made around initiating, continuing or discontinuing treatment and interpretations of the professionals conduct during sometimes intimate investigations and treatment. Although this protection is important and necessary, it sometimes benefits the members and the profession at the expense of patient safety and a number of examples in relation to the profession of medicine are now given.

Harold Shipman

The case of Harold Shipman, the English GP convicted of multiple murder, is the most dramatic and saddest case of threats to patient safety that can be attributed, in part at least, to the dangers professional membership can bring. His case is relevant here because his status served to legitimise his activities and to shield him from investigation both from inside or outside medicine (Robinson, 2003). Harold Shipman was convicted on 15 counts of murder and forgery of a patient's will on the 31 January 2000. He was sentenced to life imprisonment with a recommendation from the judge that he never be released. He murdered his patients by administering large doses of opiates (some sedatives were also probably used), usually diamorphine (Smith, 2005). Shipman committed suicide whilst in prison in 2004. His activities, and the investigations they led to, have given rise to changes to healthcare practice in the NHS that will enhance patient safety.

Two different methods of calculating the numbers of patients he murdered were completed. The first was a retrospective audit of his general practice including an analysis of death certificates issued by him between 1974 and 1998. It included comparisons with GPs with similar workloads and concluded that there were 236 excess deaths about which there should be concern (Baker, 2001). The second calculation was reached through the public inquiry into the extent of his unlawful activity. This culminated in the publication of six extensive reports (Smith 2002; 2003; 2003a; 2004; 2004a; 2005) that traced his career from medical school through to his arrest in 1998 for the murder of Mrs Grudy and forgery of her will. The calculation in the Smith inquiry of the number of murders committed was very similar to the result reached in the Baker (2001) audit, even though very different methods were used. In the final paragraph from the sixth and last of the inquiries Dame Janet Smith summarises the position thus.

'f I were to assume that 50% of the deaths that I regarded as suspicious were in fact unlawful killings, my estimate for the Todmorden and Hyde years would come to 237 or 238, very close indeed to Professor Baker's estimate. That being so, it seems to me not unreasonable to take Professor Baker's figure as the most reliable estimate of the number of unlawful killings during these two periods. If I then add in my estimate of unlawful killings in Pontefract, I arrive at a total of about 250 deaths. My overall conclusion is that Shipman killed about 250 patients between 1971 and 1998, of whom I have been able positively to identify 218'

Smith, 2005: 101

Harold Shipman was therefore murdering people for many years, yet little suspicion about his activities was raised either by the public, other healthcare workers or the systems and organisations within which he worked (Smith, 2002).

Comment from those in the local community showed that many people had their suspicions about his activities but felt unable to report them. For example, a local taxi driver was concerned because his regular fares, the elderly ladies he took shopping and to the post office to collect their pension, were dying in significant numbers if they were Shipman's patients (Whittle and Ritchie, 2000). The routine nature of these trips meant that he, and his wife who kept a list of clients, knew the women well and the link with Shipman became clear due to the visits to the GP that elderly people often make. Similarly, the local undertaker noticed that many of Shipman's patients died with their clothes on sitting up in a chair. This is unusual in elderly people who suffer a medical crisis and die at home. These crises commonly include a heart attack or stroke and the person will therefore end up on the floor, or the event occurs whilst they are in bed or on the toilet. As with the taxi driver and his wife, the undertaker's staff felt unable to say anything about their concerns. They doubted their own judgement on the matter, and they doubted that anyone would listen to them if they queried the activities of a professional, especially one who was so well known locally (Whittle and Ritchie, 2000).

Shipman's relationship with drug therapy was a complex one in which he appeared at times to test and push the boundaries of drug dosages on patients (Smith, 2002; Smith, 2005). He had previously been addicted to the synthetic opiate pethidine and particular attention was paid to this period of his career in the fifth report of the inquiry (Smith, 2004a). It was estimated that he had taken over 83,000 milligrams of pethidine before his dismissal from the general practice in Todmorden, Yorkshire. An average adult dose for pain relief (it is only used for the relief of moderate to severe pain) is 50 to 100 milligrams, usually no more than four times a day. Shipman admitted to the police that he was injecting 600 to 700 milligrams of pethidine a day at the height of his addiction (Whittle and Ritchie, 2000). One unlawful and six suspicious deaths were subsequently attributed to Shipman for 1975, the year before his convictions for the misuse of pethidine (Peters, 2005).

In 1976 his case in relation to the pethidine addiction was referred to the Penal Cases Committee of the General Medical Council (GMC), the regulatory body for the medical profession in the UK. Shipman had been convicted of dishonestly obtaining a controlled drug by deception, forgery of NHS prescriptions and unlawful possession of a controlled drug. He asked for 74 similar offences to be taken into consideration (Smith, 2004a). The Penal Cases Committee, which sat in private, considered his case but decided not to refer the matter on to the Disciplinary Committee. The latter had the power to either suspend medical staff for up to a year or erase the name of the practitioner from the professional register. The Penal Cases Committee had no such powers and simply gave him a warning leaving him free to practice medicine unrestricted.

These events raise the question, what did a doctor have to do to be referred to the Disciplinary Committee? This was addressed in the Shipman Inquiry and it seemed that if medical staff with drug addictions, and Dame Janet Smith (2004a) noted it was not (and probably is still not) an uncommon problem, sought psychiatric help and responded to that help the Penal Cases Committee were unlikely to refer the matter on. The outcome of the Penal Cases Committee decision meant that during the application process for his next post in 1977 no mention was made by the GMC of his previous conviction for pethidine addiction. Dame Janet Smith (2004a) was highly critical of the GMC on this point and suggested that any restrictions that are placed on a doctors record (none were placed on Shipman's record) should be available to the public. The GMC has now updated its online search facility and a doctor's registration can be checked by the public, along with any restrictions that might be in place (go to www.gmc-uk.org). Shipman did admit to his addiction when applying for the new post in 1977, but played down the severity of the situation. In 1992 he was able to set up as a single-handed GP, a position that reduced the chances of his on-going criminal activity being detected.

With regard to the regulation and procedures for use of diamorphine in the community the systems were so slack that in at least six cases Shipman was able to write prescriptions for the drug even though the patient was already dead! Dame Janet Smith (2004, p6) noted: "Between 1992 and 1998, Shipman obtained more that 24,000 milligans of diamorphine illicitly. During that time, he killed 143 patients and I am suspicious about a further nine deaths". Controls and audit on the use of opiates in the community have been revised and strengthened in response to the Shipman inquiry and further changes to legislation in this area are in process (Clinical Governance Support Team et al, 2005; HM Government, 2005). Similarly, the process for issuing death certificates is under review at the time of writing with the possibility of new legislation being introduced although there appears to be a lack of consensus on the way forward at the time of writing (see Secretary of State for Constitutional Affairs and Lord Chancellor, 2006). Changes were made to the cremation certification process in England, Wales and Northern Ireland following publication of a fundamental review of the death certification process, known as the Luce report (Secretary of State for the Home Department, 2003). A doctor asked to sign the second part of a cremation certificate is now obliged to speak to a person who had contact with the patient before their death. This change should increase the possibility of the public raising concerns over a death if they felt it was suspicious.

Peter Green

The case of Harold Shipman is a unique, it is hoped, and extreme example of the harm that can occur when professionals abuse their position and the profession and the systems within which the professional work fail to detect and/or act on that abuse. However, other examples of malicious practice exist and we now move on to the case of Peter Green.

In July 2000 Peter Green, a GP from Loughborough, England, was convicted on nine counts of indecent assault on five patients. He had originally been charged on seventeen counts of indecent assault, one of which involved a minor patient. The conviction was the culmination of concerns raised over a period of 12 years and followed three separate police inquiries. The investigation completed by the Commission for Healthcare Improvement (2001) found that between 1985 and 1997 a number of patients had tried to raise concerns with the family health service authority, other doctors at the practice, the police and officers of the General Medical Council (GMC). The patients complaints related to the conduct of Peter Green during consultations.

It was not until June 1997 following concerns raised by a health visitor that positive action ensued. The local medical director to whom the complaint was made contacted Leicestershire Health Authority and the story began to unfold with the matter being referred to the GMC Fitness to Practice Directorate in July 1997. As the GMC investigation took some time to proceed, and the health authority did not have the power to suspend Green, his partners at the surgery, on taking legal advice, had to dissolve the practice. This did not stop Green continuing to practice. He, like Shipman, became a single-handed practitioner and also a member of the out-of-hours service, positions he was able to hold for a further eight months. He was eventually suspended from the medical register in June 1998 pending the outcome of the criminal inquiry described above. The Commission for Healthcare Improvement (2001) investigation was critical of the time it took the GMC to take action. The GMC was also described as 'sluggish' in its response by some of those who gave evidence to the investigation.

Rather like Shipman, Green was able to misuse a 'prescription only medication' for his own purposes, in this case midazolam, a sedating agent that is associated with memory loss. He sexually assaulted male patients whilst they were under the influence of the drug (Commission for Healthcare Improvement, 2001). The investigation concluded that a culture existed in the NHS that did not listen to, or treat complaints inquisitively allowing:

> '*...a credible person to do incredible things to patients to whom he had a duty of care*'
>> Commission for Healthcare Improvement, 2001: vii original emphasis

Acknowledgment of the potential value of complaints as a means of enhancing patient safety is gathering momentum. This notion is explored in a chapter by Burke (2003) that analysed the now defunct Community Health Councils contribution to patient safety and is evident in at least two National Patient Safety Agency initiatives. The first is the attempt to establish an 'open and fair' culture in the NHS (NPSA, 2005) and the second is the facility for public reporting of patient safety incidents (www.npsa.nhs.uk/pleaseask). This is a significant step forward in patient safety as this frees the patient to report incidents without having to encounter the barriers that can be put in their way by healthcare staff and/or the bureaucratic systems within which they seek to raise a concern. The same web site offers the public the opportunity to register a compliant if they so wish.

Richard Neale

Moving on now from examples of malicious practice, we turn to the problem of inept practitioners. Richard Neale attained full registration with the GMC in 1971. After working in the UK as a GP for a short period of time he moved to Canada. In 1978, whilst practicing in British Columbia, he performed a high-risk operation against the advice of a more senior colleague, which resulted in the patient's death. Following an investigation he lost his hospital privileges and was required to either undergo further training or cease practice. He did complete further training and moved to Ontario where, in 1981, another investigation was initiated into the treatment he administered to a woman during childbirth. The woman died from a massive amniotic fluid emboli after her womb ruptured, a complication directly attributed in the subsequent investigation to his treatment. In 1985 his name was erased from the Canadian Medical Register following a disciplinary hearing that found his actions in relation to the handling of this women's case had been incompetent and amounted to serious professional misconduct (DH, 2004a). The disciplinary hearing concluded that

Neale's attitude to some patients and colleagues was arrogant, dismissive and overbearing thus stifling the possibility of complaints by patients and criticisms by colleagues. He was over-confident in his descriptions of the likely outcomes of clinical interventions, was not a good communicator and was often unduly optimistic when giving patients a prognosis. Neale had resigned from the College of Physicians and Surgeons of Ontario before the hearing sat. He did not attend or send representation to the hearing and, as a result of these events, left Canada and returned to the United Kingdom to work in the NHS. On return to the UK he applied for and gained a consultant gynaecologist post in Northallerton, Yorkshire. He subsequently tried to regain registration in Canada on a number of occasions but failed.

An independent investigation was initiated in 2002 (DH, 2004a) to ascertain how allegations about Neale's performance and conduct were handled by the NHS and the relevant professional bodies. The inquiry was initiated in response to public concern over Neale being allowed to practice, both in the NHS and private sector in the UK when concerns about his honesty and ability had been raised for many years and he had been struck off in Canada. The chairman of the inquiry judged that there were serious systems failures in the employment and complaints procedures of the NHS:

> '...and very importantly, failures within other professional bodies upon whom the NHS were dependent'
>
> Department of Health, 2004a: 13

The significance of complaints procedures, and as with other cases mentioned here complaints against Neale were often not listened to or acted upon, was mentioned earlier in this chapter so the discussion here moves on to the two professional bodies implicated in the chairman's comments. They were the General Medical Council (GMC) and the British Medical Association (BMA).

The General Medical Council was notified by two separate routes in 1985 that Neale had been 'struck off' in Canada. The GMC representative at the independent investigation (DH, 2004a) initially denied that they had been informed of this in 1985/6 by the police but subsequently had to accept that this had happened when irrefutable police evidence was brought forward. These notifications and the serious events that occurred in Canada did not stop Neale registering with the GMC to practice in the UK as a consultant gynaecologist. Complaints about his performance continued to be raised and an earlier and smaller inquiry had been launched in 1993 by the hospital Trust for which he worked; the Peterson Investigation. Papers available to this investigation included, amongst others, details of the Canadian incidents that led to Neale being first cautioned and then struck off, and a police caution related to an incident in some public toilets. Neale had previously tried to gain a position as a police surgeon and specialist in sex cases, yet he was cautioned in 1991 for allegedly watching two homosexuals indulging in a sex act in a public toilet in Richmond. When questioned by the police he denied the allegation and stated he was in the toilet to eat his lunch! He accepted a verbal caution from the police (DH, 2004a).

The British Medical Association (BMA), the professional association for doctors, were highly protective of Neale in relation to the Peterson investigation. In a letter to the investigation team they made it clear that the BMA did not accept the terms of reference of the investigation. Indeed, they suggested that the Trust should be making a public statement of support for Richard Neale, not investigating him. They closed this letter by stating that neither they nor Richard Neale would be attending the preliminary meeting to determine the process of the investigation and added:

'It does, of course, go without saying that should the investigation proceed on 17 December 1993 we shall rigorously and robustly represent and defend Richard Neale's interests'

Department of Health, 2004: 97 original emphasis

In a further letter to the investigation team the BMA cited the European Convention on Human Rights and the UN Convention on Social and Political Rights in Neale's defence. Neale did appear before the investigation, with BMA representation, and ten recommendations were made. These limited both his public and work activities but allowed him to continue employment at the Northallerton Trust. Neale only rejected one of the recommendations, to be resident at the hospital or within a 10 mile radius from the hospital site when on call. The BMA supported his rejection on this point, even though it was intended to ensure that he, like other on-call medical staff, would be readily available if a patient needed them in an emergency — it was then a requirement imposed to try to enhance patient safety. The Committee of Inquiry found that Neale had been dishonest on this point by purchasing a house outside the 'hospital zone' — the 10 mile radius requirement.

Neale's case illustrates a number of shortcomings in professional regulation. Although processes at the GMC have changed and registration status in other countries is now taken into consideration, it is difficult to stop a professional practicing when they are insistent on doing so. As in the previous case of Peter Green, it is also difficult for healthcare staff to challenge a professional and this can again be seen in the case of Rodney Ledward, the last to be explored in detail here.

Rodney Ledward

Rodney Ledward was a gynaecologist who was struck off the UK medical register in 1998. An inquiry was initiated in 1999 on the request of the Secretary of State for Health to ascertain why the serious failures in the practice of Ledward were not identified and acted upon earlier. The inquiry was held in private but the full report, known as the Ritchie Report (2000) was made public. It describes, in chronological order, the vagaries of Ledward's practice from 1980 to 1996 and sought evidence from a wide range of documentary sources and witnesses, some of whom remained supportive of Ledward. He became unwell and was not able to appear at the inquiry. Some of the problems he created were described in the report thus:

> *'We have been made aware that many patients were caused upset, worry, and anxiety by Rodney Ledward and many were also caused physical injury. Many have been scarred physically and emotionally. Some had a physical problem which ought to have been readily capable of correction under Rodney Ledward's care, but they were caused injury or further problems. Some appear to have been subjected to repeated and unnecessary surgical procedures. Some already had both physical and emotional problems when they were referred to Rodney Ledward; it seems that his treatment exacerbated their condition'*

Ritchie Report, 2000: 14

Ledward, for financial gain, had actively encouraged many women he had treated during NHS work to become private patients. The evidence in the report suggests that this was a dangerous shift as unnecessary surgery was more common amongst his private patients:

> *'... we express our concern as to whether all these procedures were medically necessary'*

Ritchie Report, 2000: 90, original emphasis

This is a comment made by the inquiry team on a number of occasions throughout the report. Hysterectomy, removal of the womb, was one such procedure which he often performed on comparatively young women.

What is particularly sad when reading the Ritchie Report, like the other cases mentioned here, is the length of time it took for the vagaries of his practice to become public. Each of the three main sections of the report spans a period of about five years yet they contain similar concerns with regard to his practice. One of the significant issues in the Ledward case was the division between his private practice and NHS work. To each set of staff he appeared to be an unfortunate or unlucky surgeon who ran into more than his fair share of problems. If the two sets of staff had been aware that the same types of problems were occurring in the other sector, then the alarm with regard to Leward's practice might have been raised earlier. Rather ironically, both

Richard Neale and Rodney Ledward were involved in work relating to medical audit, an integral part of the clinical governance agenda.

Summary of Patient Safety Lessons

These and other cases, for example the Kerr/Haslam Inquiry (HM Government, 2005a) from the mental health setting, illustrate some of the threats to patient safety that professional status and ineffective organisational processes can create. Examples from medicine have been focused on here as medicine meets the criteria of a profession. There are many other examples, and Repper (1995) completed a literature review on healthcare practitioners who were considered to be exhibiting symptoms of Munchausen Syndrome by Proxy. This is a situation in which the perpetrator induces symptoms, sometimes life threatening, in another person (the patient when it occurs in healthcare practitioners). This is done in an attempt to demonstrate, in a covert fashion, how effective the care and treatment they can give is when the victim is taken ill. The most important case in the UK was the enrolled nurse Beverley Allitt who killed or severely injured 13 children in the hospital setting by injecting high doses of insulin (Clothier, 1994).

If a practitioner is malicious then they will, by definition, do what they can to avoid detection. Similarly, the inept or incompetent practitioner is probably not self-aware with regard to the limits of their practice and may therefore evade detection. It is almost certainly not possible to stop all such cases occurring in the future, but healthcare systems need to become more efficient at detecting and acting upon such behaviour. The changes described above, made to opiate regulation in the community setting and cremation certification, are examples of such change and followed the Harold Shipman case. In human factors theory it is accepted that error cannot be completely eradicated, but you can reduce the number and severity of those errors. The same would hold true here with regard to malicious and inept professionals: we can not completely remove the risk but we can reduce the impact of their actions and detect them earlier. Professions and organisations can therefore be dysfunctional in terms of patient safety, by protecting and/or failing to detect practitioners who are malicious or who are not maintaining adequate standards. We therefore need to be 'malicious and inept-practitioner wary' within our own practice.

Professional Regulation and Organisational Management

The cases cited above demonstrate that professional status and regulation along with organisational management are crucial factors in patient safety. They are inevitably a key part of any attempt to create the learning environment described by Duffy and Saul (2003) earlier in this chapter. In the UK the emphasis placed on healthcare professions and organisations within the context of the patient safety agenda, has increased since the instigation of clinical governance. The GMC (2005) in its 'vision for the future' document claims it has made, and will continue to make, significant changes in its mechanisms acknowledging that many of these changes are in response to cases such as those reviewed in this chapter. The GMC has achieved greater patient/public involvement and has made registration more meaningful and accessible to the public. Public involvement has also increased with a forty percent lay representation on the GMC Council. One of the identified themes to improve future regulation at the GMC is 'making sense of complaints', and the importance of this is clearly illustrated within this chapter. Healthcare professionals need to view complainants as allies in the task of improving patient safety: they need to be invited into what Hughes' (1993) called the 'charmed circle' of professions, and be encouraged to actively participate in their care and treatment.

Like the GMC, there have also been changes at the Nursing and Midwifery Council (NMC) that reflect pressures felt from the patient safety agenda. On taking over from the United Kingdom Central Council and the four National Boards in 2002, a Conduct and Competence Committee was added to the two that already existed: the Professional Conduct Committee and Health Committee. This new emphasis on competence, created through the Nursing and Midwifery Order 2001 (NMC, 2004), reflects some of the problems described in the cases given in this chapter and demonstrates a toughening of NMC expectations on nurse/midwife performance in practice. At the time of writing the NMC proficiencies that guide curriculum development are also under review. As the core purpose of the NMC is 'protecting the public through professional standards' (go to www.nmc-uk.org) it is hoped that clearer references to patient safety will be evident in the revised proficiencies.

Another recent development in terms of professional regulation was the creation of the Council for Healthcare Regulatory Excellence (CHRE). This came into being in 2003 in part response to the Kennedy report (Kennedy et al, 2000), the aspect of the Bristol inquiry that dealt with the scandal that arose around issues of consent and the removal of organs from babies at post-mortem. The Report called for a reconnection between regulated professions and the public. The CHRE focuses on fitness for purpose and has a co-ordinating function that promotes the interests of the public and best practice in regulating healthcare professionals (CHRE, 2003). Its work covers nine different professions in health care including the GMC and the NMC. Its existence is evidence of the professional predicament faced by healthcare groups as it is a challenge to the historical authority of professions, particularly medicine, drawing these different healthcare professions together under one authority. In the 2004/5 report and accounts of the CHRE it is noted that the organisation successfully appealed eight cases to court that it considered had be too leniently dealt with by a professional body (CHRE, 2005). In 2005/6 the figure rose slightly to ten cases (CHRE, 2006). The CHRE appeals cases to the high court and the majority of these are upheld. Would some of the cases mentioned in this chapter have been subject to such referral if the CHRE, or an equivalent, had been in existence?

Another repercussion from the Bristol Royal Infirmary Inquiry was the creation of a code of conduct for NHS managers (DH, 2002a). Its purpose is to guide managers in the decision making process and reassure the public that accountability is in place. The first principle stated in the code obliges the manager to make the care and safety of patients their first priority. Specific mention is also made of processes to ensure that appropriate support for staff and disciplinary procedures are in place. This code, like the creation of the CHRE and the changes described at the NMC, shows a common motivational focus in terms of its origins – patient safety. The cases illustrated here, along with the many others that have not been described, have helped to shift health care towards a culture of patient safety.

Multidisciplinary Working

The examples of malicious and inept practice given above show some of the threats to patient safety that occur, in part at least, due to inadequacies within professional regulation and organisational bureaucracy. Turning again to lessons learnt from safety critical industries, team working, what I will refer to as multidisciplinary working in the health care context, is emphasised as being central to the development and maintenance of a safety culture. However, it can be seen from the brief analysis given of professions above that team working is not a trait of professions; the profession seeks to define and boundary its work for its 'charmed circle' of members (Hughes, 1993). Effective team working also relies on power sharing amongst the team members but the very nature of professional groups leads to an element of competition. Which group is the more powerful? This creates an exclusivity that impedes rather than facilitates team working. This is made evident in health care through the power advantage that medicine holds, what Wicks (1998) calls a discourse of domination in her research into the shifting nature of doctor/nurse boundaries. Wicks also notes that this relationship is a problematic one for nursing as, unlike other occupational groups in health care, it is historically grafted to medicine. The work of the Council for Healthcare Regulatory Excellence (CHRE) does, in the context of professional regulation, bring various professional groups together. Bearing in mind the characteristics of a profession described in the opening of the chapter, the CHRE does challenge the historical power individual professions have sought to wield.

Going back to a point raised earlier in the chapter, with regard to health care needing to learn from other industries, research has shown that when compared to aviation staff, senior medical staff are more likely to deny the detrimental effects of fatigue and are less likely to listen to the views of juniors (Sexton et al, 2000). Although emergency work is an inevitable response to some healthcare needs, for example emergency surgery, the reluctance of medicine to accept human fallibility in relation to otherwise well understood psychological concepts, such as fatigue, is increasingly baffling. The Sexton research also showed that listening and taking advice from those outside the profession was difficult for medical staff. This is relevant for nurses who will often guide and influence medical staff during the treatment and prescription processes. This has been referred to as the 'Doctor nurse' game and has been explored elsewhere in relation to the use of thrombolytic drugs in acute myocardial infarction (Flisher and Burns, 2003). One of the important points made by Flisher and Burn is that what matters, in terms of the effective and safe management of these patients in the acute treatment phase, is the knowledge and skill the practitioner has, not their professional orientation. Although the 'doctor nurse' game feels less relevant in today's healthcare system, the lesson of open and fair working remains. Staff that feel able to freely communicate and share ideas and responsibilities within an effective team working system are likely to be more effective practitioners (Vincent, 2006). As healthcare staff we need to think critically about professional boundaries and whether they are impinging on patient safety.

Conclusion

As outlined at the start of this chapter, patient safety is a new agenda that allows us to more clearly focus upon the unnecessary harm, errors and malicious and inept practice that has often been hidden within the daily work of health care. It is an agenda that will facilitate significant improvements in the quality of care and treatment. It is also, however, an agenda that brings challenges. If the goal of health care is the promotion of health then anything that challenges that goal is worthy of scrutiny and this holds true with regard to concepts such as professional status and organisational structure and processes. We cannot and should not assume as healthcare practitioners that organisational and bureaucratic factors are not our concern. They are because, like professional regulation, they can enhance or adversely affect patient safety. Only a comparatively small number of patient safety incidents can be attributed to malicious and inept practice, yet as the cases analysed here show, these cases can and do have a profound effect on many people.

It has been argued here that some patient safety incidents are directly attributable to professional status, especially in relation to the work of medicine. Aspects of this harm are also due to systems failures within the bureaucracy of organisational work. More rarely that harm is due to malicious and inept practice. The evidence cited here shows that it is reasonable for the public to be concerned about the abilities of professions and healthcare organisations to protect their safety. Such wariness is perhaps in itself healthy, although this adds an additional worry to those that patients bring with them when using health services. A key purpose of professional regulation is to maintain and where possible enhance standards of practice and personal conduct so that the patient feels able to trust the practitioner. If the concept of trust is seen to embrace sharing knowledge, and greater patient participation and partnership, then the trend towards patients taking more responsibility is, literally speaking, healthy and good for patient safety. Active patient participation is a challenge to the historical superiority of medicine in health care, as is multi-disciplinary working. Yet these changes, what might be considered by some as threats to professional integrity, are required to enhance patient safety.

Key points in the professional role in patient safety:

- Accept that improving patient safety is a priority and an avenue through which the nations health can be significantly improved
- Be error and systems aware
- Report patient safety incidents, including near miss events, and continue to enhance the quality of that reporting
- Actively engage with patient safety initiatives at a personal, local and national level. The latter is possible through the active and detailed reporting of patient safety incidents
- Put the patient first, not the profession, fellow professionals or the organisation
- Encourage patients to use complaints procedures and/or the patient safety incident reporting system now in place
- Facilitate the generation of an open and fair culture in healthcare
- Be malicious- and inept-practitioner wary.

I would like to thank Professor Kate Robinson, University of Bedfordshire, for her guidance on aspects of this chapter.

References

Arah OA, Klazinga NS (2004) How safe is the safety paradigm? *Qual Saf Health Care* **13**(3): 226-232

Baker R (2001) *Harold Shipman's Clinical Practice 1974-1998*. Department of Health, London

Brennan TA, Leape LL, Laird NM et al (1991) Incidence of adverse events and negligence in hospitalized patients. Results of the Harvard Medical Practice Study I. *N Engl J Med* **324**: 370-376

Bristol Royal Infirmary Inquiry (2001) *Learning from Bristol. The Report of the Public Inquiry into Children's Heart Surgery at the Bristol Royal Infirmary, 1984-1995*. Department of Health, London

Burke A (2003) Complaints as a measure of harm — lessons from Community Health Councils. In: Milligan F J, Robinson K (eds). *Limiting Harm in Health Care: A Nursing Perspective*. Blackwell Science, Oxford

Clinical Governance Support Team, National Patient Safety Agency, National Clinical Assessment Service and Royal Pharmaceutical Society of Great Britain (2005) *Clinical Governance Toolkit for Controlled Drug Management in Primary Care in the NHS*. Clinical Governance Support Team, Leicester

Clothier C (1994) *The Independent Inquiry Relating to Deaths and Injuries on the Children's Ward at Grantham and Kesteven Hospital during the period February to April 1991*. HMSO, London

Commission for Healthcare Improvement (2001) *Investigation into Issues Arising from the Case of Loughborough GP Peter Green*. CHI, London

Comptroller and Auditor General (2004) *Improving Patient Care by Reducing the Risk of Hospital Acquired Infection: A Progress Report*. National Audit Office, London

Comptroller and Auditor General (2005) *A Safer Place for Patients: Learning to Improve Patient Safety*. National Audit Office, London

Council for Healthcare Regulatory Excellence (2003) *Council for Healthcare Regulatory Excellence. What We Do*. CHRE, London

Council for Healthcare Regulatory Excellence (2005) *Annual Report and Accounts 2004/5*. The Stationery Office, London

Council for Healthcare Regulatory Excellence (2006) *Annual Report and Summary Accounts 2005/6*. The Stationery Office, London

Davies C (1995) *Gender and the Professional Predicament in Nursing*. Open University Press, Buckingham

DH (2000) *An Organisation with a Memory. Report of an expert group on learning from adverse events in the NHS chaired by the Chief medical Officer*. The Stationary Office, London

DH (2001) *Building a Safer NHS for Patients: implementing An Organisation with a Memory*. The Stationary Office, London

DH (2002) *Learning from Bristol: the Department of Health's Response to the Report of the Public Inquiry into Children's Heart Surgery at the Bristol Royal infirmary 1984-1995.* The Stationary Office, London

DH (2002a) *Code of Conduct for NHS Managers.* DH, London

DH (2004) *Standards for Better Health.* DH, London

DH (2004a) *Committee of Inquiry to Investigate how the NHS Handled Allegations about the Performance and Conduct of Richard Neale.* The Stationery Office, Norwich

Department for Transport (2004) *Road casualties in Great Britain: 2003.* Transport Statistics Publications, London

Duffy RB, Saull JW (2003) *Know the Risk. Learning from Errors and Accidents: safety and risk in today's technology.* Butterworth Heinemann, Amsterdam

Flisher D, Burns M (2003) Nurse diagnosed myocardial infarction – hidden nurse work and iatrogenic risk. In: Milligan FJ, Robinson K, eds. *Limiting Harm in Health Care: A Nursing Perspective.* Blackwell Science, Oxford, p171-193

General Medical Council (2005) *Developing Medical Regulation: a Vision for the Future.* General Medical Council, London

HM Government (2005) *Safer Management of controlled drugs. The Government's response to the fourth report of the Shipman inquiry.* The Stationery Office, Norwich

HM Government (2005a) *The Kerr/Haslam Inquiry.* The Stationery Office, Norwich

Hughes E C (1993) License and mandate. In: Walmsley J, Reynolds J, Shakespeare P, Woolfe R (eds) *Health Welfare and Practice.* Sage, London: 21-31

Kennedy I, Howard R, Jarman B, Maclean M (2000) *The inquiry into the management of care of children receiving complex heart surgery at The Bristol Royal Infirmary. Interim report — removal and retention of human material.* The Bristol Royal Infirmary, Bristol

Kohn LT, Corrigan JM, Donaldson MS (eds) (2000) *To Err is human: building a safer health system.* National Academy Press, Washington D.C

Leape LL, Brennan TA, Laird NM et al (1991) The nature of adverse events in hopsitalized patients. Results of the Harvard Medical Practice study II. *N Engl J Med* **324**: 377-384

Leape L (1999) Error in medicine. In: Rosenthal M M, Mulcahy L, Lloyd-Bostock S (eds) *Medical mishaps; pieces of the puzzle.* Open University Press, Buckingham: 20-38

Milligan FJ (2003) Defining medicine and the nature of iatrogenic harm. In: Milligan FJ, Robinson K (eds) *Limiting harm in health care: a nursing perspective.* Blackwell Science, Oxford

Milligan FJ, Robinson K (eds) (2003) *Limiting harm in health care: a nursing perspective.* Blackwell Science, Oxford

NPSA (2004) *Seven Steps to Patient Safety: an overview guide for staff.* 2nd print. NPSA, London

NPSA (2005) *Safer Practice Notice. Being open when patients are harmed.* NPSA,

London

NPSA (2005a) P*atient Briefing. Being open – saying sorry when things go wrong.* NPSA, London

NPSA (2005b) *Building a memory: preventing harm, reducing risks and improving patient safety.* NPSA, London

NPSA (2006) Quarterly National Reporting and Learning System data summary. NPSA, London

National Health Performance Committee (2004) *National Report on health sector performance indicators.* Australian Institute of Health and Welfare, Canberra

NMC (2004) *Reporting lack of competence: a guide for employers and managers.* NMC, London

Peters C (2005) *Harold Shipman. Mind set on murder.* Sevenoaks, London

Repper J (1995) Munchausen syndrome by proxy in health care workers. *J Adv Nurs* **21**(2): 299-304

Reason J (2004) Beyond the organisational accident: the need for 'error wisdom' on the front line. *Qual Saf Health Care Supp* **2**: ii 28-33

Ritchie Report (2000) *Report of the inquiry into quality and practice within the National Health Service arising from the actions of Rodney Ledward.* DH, London

Robinson K (2003) Professions, power, knowledge and expertise. In: Milligan F J, Robinson K (eds) *Limiting harm in health care: a nursing perspective.* Blackwell, Science Oxford

Savage J (1987) *Nurses gender and sexuality.* Heinemann, London

Secretary of State for the Home Department (2003) *Death certification and investigation in England, Wales and Northern Ireland. The report of a fundamental review.* The Stationery Office, Norwich

Secretary of State for Constitutional Affairs and Lord Chancellor (2006) *Reform of the Coroners' System and Death Certification: Government Response to the Constitutional Affairs Select Committee's Report.* Stationery Office, Norwich

Sexton JB, Thomas EJ, Helmreich RL (2000) Error, stress, and teamwork in medicine and aviation: cross sectional surveys. *Br Med J* **320**: 745-749

Sharpe VA, Faden AI (1998) *Medical harm; historical, conceptual, ethical dimensions of iatrogenic illness.* Cambridge University Press, Cambridge

Smith J (2002) *The Shipman inquiry: first report. Volume 1, death disguised.* The Shipman Inquiry, Manchester

Smith J (2003) *The Shipman inquiry: second report – The police investigation of March 1998.* The Shipman Inquiry, Manchester

Smith J (2003a) *The Shipman inquiry: third report – Death certification and the investigation of deaths by coroners.* The Shipman Inquiry, Manchester

Smith J (2004) *The Shipman inquiry - fourth report – The regulation of controlled drugs in the community.* The Shipman Inquiry, Manchester

Smith J (2004a) *The Shipman inquiry: fifth report – Safeguarding patients: lessons from the past – proposals for the future.* The Shipman Inquiry, Manchester

Smith J (2005) *The Shipman inquiry - sixth report – Shipman: the final report.* The Shipman Inquiry, Manchester

Ulich R, Quan X, Zimring C, Joseph A, Choudhary R (2004) *The role of the physical environment in the hospital of the 21st century: a once-in-a-lifetime opportunity.* Centre for Health Design, Concord CA

Vincent C, Neale G, Woloshynowych M (2001) Adverse events in British hospitals: preliminary retrospective record review. *BMJ* **322**: 517-519

Vincent C, Reason J (1999) Human factors approaches in medicine. In: Rosenthal M M, Mulcahy L, Lloyd-Bostock S (eds) *Medical mishaps; pieces of the puzzle.* Open University Press, Buckingham, p 39-56

Vincent C (2006) *Patient Safety.* Churchill Livingstone, Edinburgh

Wicks D (1998) *Nurses and doctors at work; re-thinking professional boundaries.* Open University Press, Buckingham

Wiegmann D A, Shappell S A (2003) A human error approach to aviation accident analysis. Ashgate, Aldershot

Wilson R, Runciman W B, Gibberd R W, Harrison B T, Newby L, Hamilton J D (1995) The quality in Australian health care study. *Med J Aust* **163**: 458-471

Whittle B, Ritchie J (2000) *Prescription for murder. The true story of mass murderer Dr Harold Frederick Shipman.* Warner Books, London

CHAPTER 4

The Role of the National Patient Safety Agency

Peter Mansell, Wendy Harris, Jane Carthey, Imran Haider Syed,

This chapter aims to provide readers with both the context in which greater patient and public participation in health care was born, and describe how the National Patient Safety Agency (NPSA) developed to shape to the nature of lay involvement in its work.

A number of organisations and writers have visualised a more active role for individual patients and their families in contributing to their own and others safety in healthcare (National Consumer Council, 2002; JCAHO, 2002; Vincent et al, 2002; ISMP, 2003). It is clear from the NPSA's work so far that the involvement of patients and those close to them add value in a variety of ways (NPSA, 2004) including: their reporting of incidents; sharing views of the causes and issues surrounding Patient Safety Incidents (PSIs) and helping to transform the culture of the NHS (Modernisation Agency, 2002).

Patient involvement can be distinguished from public involvement. The former refers to the involvement of individual patients and those very closely associated with their experience as patients, for example, carers and family members in decisions regarding their own health and health care. The latter refers to the involvement of members of the public in strategic decisions about national or local health service policy (Florin and Dixon, 2004).

Lay involvement is often used as a general term and can refer to a range of participation — see *Table 4.1*. Choices about who to involve are linked to the nature of the issue in question. For example, the NPSA could just involve its lay board members. However, that would not provide the Agency with the diversity of voices it needs to hear in order to make health care safer.

How Patients Understand Safety

The Reporting Gap

The NHS is one of the largest healthcare providers in the world (DH, 2000a) and the likelihood of individuals coming to serious harm, for example, dying or

Table 4.1. Types of participants		
Who	Types of participation - from individual to representative	
Patient	Individual experience of error and harm	Individual experience that is used to relate to and represent common themes
Patient representative	Individual experiences of services	
Carer		
Member of the public	Individual perceptions	
Interest group	Collective experiences used to draw out common themes in related areas	

being permanently disabled as a result of a patient safety incident is remote. For example, a typical primary care organisation (e.g. a group of GP surgeries covering a population of 250,000) may experience 11,500 consultation errors, 7,000 of which would be preventable in a year. A typical acute hospital (500 beds) may experience 3,500 patient safety incidents, of which 1,700 would be preventable. While estimates do vary, the evidence of harm in hospitals suggests that up to 70,000 people may suffer injury as a result of a patient safety incident, half of which may be preventable (Vincent et al, 2001; NPSA, 2005a).

Research and current trends in reporting (NPSA, 2005a) show that patient safety incidents are not limited to just a few tragic high profile incidents. Because the NHS is so large the data translates into massive (tens of thousands) of numbers. This means that the NHS pays high mitigation and compensation costs in relation to errors (£450million in 2002) (DH, 2003a). Yet evidence suggests there is massive under-reporting (Cullen et al, 1995; Barach and Small, 2000; Weingart et al, 2000; Lawton and Parker, 2002) and the NPSA believes that one of the key reasons for this is fear by clinicians that reporting errors will not lead to improved safety rather it will result in their being scapegoated (Kingston et al, 2004; Waring, 2005).

Are Patients Litigious?

Patients have been a trusting group. For example, in 2000-01 there were only 140,000 formal complaints about NHS services (DH, 2003b). During September 2003 and August 2004 only 10,422 complaints were made to the Independent Complaints Advocacy Service (ICAS) (DH, 2004a) in a system where 13.5m people saw a consultant for the first time: approximately 270m consultations took place in general practice; 15.5m visited A&E; and staggering 668m prescriptions were issued in England and Wales (DH, 2004b). From these figures we can see that only a few people complain, although a small proportion (but a high actual number) of people get hurt as a result of using NHS services.

A New Approach

The Kennedy Report (Kennedy, 2001) inquiry, which began in late 1998, examined the management of the care of children receiving complex cardiac surgical services at the Bristol Royal Infirmary between 1984 and 1995. The inquiry team were charged with making findings as to the adequacy of the services provided and to make recommendations which could help to secure high quality care across the NHS.

The Bristol Report made 198 recommendations in all, with all but two recommendations (Kennedy, 2001) being accepted by the Government. These recommendations have engendered the most far-reaching structural reform and modernisation of the NHS (DH, 2001a). Such reform is expressly intended to bring the monitoring, commissioning and accountability for healthcare services closer to local people. Patient and Public Involvement (PPI) was, and is, explicitly prioritised as both a structural and a cultural driver of the new NHS.

However, the extent to which 'real' engagement has been achieved since Bristol has been contested and it has been claimed that, the NHS remains a predominately paternalistic system dominated by professional values and over-centralised control (Coulter, 2002). Accordingly, patients now use a system whose institutions and governance bodies are changing from ones that in the past have appeared closed and paternalistic to emerging institutions and governance bodes that may be more transparent, accountable and trustworthy (DH, 1998; DH, 2000a; DH, 2000b; DH, 2001b).

It was as a direct result of recommendations made in the Kennedy report that the National Patient Safety Agency (NPSA) was established (Kennedy, 2001).

Conceptualising Participation and Involvement

The NPSA was established as a Special Health Authority in July 2001, and by May 2002 the Board had decided that patients would be at heart of the its work and recruited its first Director for Patient Experience and Public Involvement (PEPI). This meant that the two key corporate sources of decision making — the NPSA's Management Team and Board – would have a member dedicated to patient and public perspectives.

By the end of 2002 it was clear that NPSA's PEPI strategy was being shaped not only by the policies mentioned above but also by the growing literature on patient and public involvement and the experiential learning from the field; the 'communities of practice' professionals, managers, 'front-line' staff, carers, and patients, all of whom are learning to work and learn together.

A key consideration was the need to develop a framework to help patients and those close to them, the public and healthcare staff, to initiate, sustain and develop successful involvement strategies that both met the spirit and letter of the Kennedy recommendations while simultaneously being as workable and as effective as possible. This led, in June 2002, to the NPSA's Board agreeing the following principles (NPSA, 2002):

- The NPSA will involve patients, service users, carers and the public
- All reasonable adjustments will be implemented to ensure participation of people with different needs can be met including the paying of fees and expenses of members of the public and participation by small organisations
- The NPSA will go beyond a simple consumer model where users are offered very limited fixed choices already determined by staff
- The NPSA acknowledges that it is not the single centre of excellence for patient safety and will strive to work closely with other places of experience, drawing knowledge from — and supporting — their work in the safety area
- Professional evidence will not be the sole criterion for NPSA activities. NPSA will recognise and act upon patient and public perceptions and experience of services to make such services both safer and as accessible as possible
- The NPSA will listen to all of its stakeholders and will avoid being dominated by any single interest
- The NPSA recognises that it will need to make difficult decisions but will retain a degree of independence from stakeholders to enable it to take such decisions.

With these principles establishing the NPSA's approach, we began to involve lay participants in a variety of ways on a number of projects, including work on infusion pumps and operational areas such as the National Reporting and Learning System (NRLS) and Business Plan, as well as developing a conceptual framework to enable staff to effectively implement lay participation.

Table 4.2 has been adapted from the various models used by the NPSA and categorises the levels of involvement adopted and used by the NPSA to help patients and staff conceptualise and assess the level and nature of involvement activities.

Involving Patients in Safety

There are three main foci for patient involvement within NPSA:

- Reporting patient safety incidents (PSIs) to the NPSA
- Shaping NPSA corporate products and activities
- Developing solutions that reduce the likelihood of harm occurring.

The methods of recruitment and specific focus of participation are determined in part by the activity, timescale any project has to undertake its work, the

Table 4.2: The Inform, Consult, Involve, Collaborate Tool			
Inform	**Consult**	**Involve**	**Collaborate**
Public participation goals			
To provide the public with balanced and objective information to assist them in understanding the problems, alternatives and/or solutions	To obtain public feedback on analysis, alternatives and/or decision	To work directly with the public throughout the process to ensure that public issues and concerns are consistently understood and considered	To partner with the public in each aspect of the decision including the development of alternatives and the identification of the preferred solution
Promise to the public			
We will keep you informed	We will keep you informed, listen to and acknowledge concerns and provide feedback on how public input influenced the decision	We will work with you to ensure that your concerns and issues are directly reflected in the alternatives developed and provide feedback on how public input influenced the decision	We will look to you for direct advice and innovation in formulating solutions and incorporate your advice and recommendations into the decision to the maximum extent possible

level of resource available to support patient involvement, and the skills of those involved. Because the NPSA (rightly) focused on making an impact on safety issues, even before it had developed its patient safety incident reporting, learning system 'solutions' work was one of the first areas for patients and those close them to become involved.

Developing Solutions

The primary method of recruitment for work on safety solutions projects has been with patients and those close to them. Once the area of a safety project has been identified, the profiles of patients at risk of harm are identified; a search of charities is completed via the Charity Commission register and letters sent to those charities working with and for people fitting the profiles. These letters alert charities to the project and invite them to express an interest in getting involved in two ways. First, the charity is invited to participate directly to use its knowledge and experience of patients' issues to bear on the project. Second, the charity acts as a both a channel of communication and recruitment and alerts its constituents the project and invites them to become involved.

Being Inclusive
This is usually done by letter and then followed up by phone or e-mail. The letters always state that the NPSA would take any reasonable steps to accommodate peoples' differing needs such as meeting carers' costs or paying for an interpreter.

In addition, the NPSA pays all expenses and often pays small allowances to thank the people for participating. This method allows NPSA to gain the involvement of those whose profiles most closely fit any given project and prevents the NPSA from becoming dominated by any one group. An example is provided below.

Example: Anticoagulation
In February of 2003, NPSA's Safe Medication Practice Team identified that the level of PSIs associated with people taking anticoagulants was high.

Across the UK 500,000 patients take anticoagulation medication (warfarin and other oral anticoagulants, and heparin by injection or infusion). Data and research (Cousins and Harris, 2003) have indicated that in primary care this group of drugs was one of the 3 most commonly associated with fatal medication errors, and in secondary care the drugs were also amongst the most frequently reported in medication errors. To use these medicines safely their dose needs to be adjusted to maintain the desired action; under-anticoagulation can result in thrombosis (which is life threatening) and over-anticoagulation can result in haemorrhage (which can also be fatal). The commonest clinical indications for the use of oral anticoagulants are atrial fibrillation, the treatment of deep vein thrombosis and pulmonary embolus, and treatment of patients with mechanical heart valves. The patients who receive anticoagulants frequently have complex medical histories and may take many other medicines. Many of the patients are also frail and elderly. Anticoagulants interact with a wide range of medicines (many commonly used such as antibiotics and analgesics). Moreover the data showed that some patient groups are more likely to experience PSIs than others, for example

- Heavy drinkers of alcohol
- People who did not administer the drug for themselves. For example, children or people living in care homes
- Those over 70 years old
- Those new to taking the drug
- Those for whom English is not their first language.

The process resulted in the first search identifying 356 charities, but many of these were found to be unsuitable as they were religious charities with the keyword Heart in their name but nothing to do with people meeting the profiles of at risk patients. Once these were removed, NPSA had 156 charities and contacted all of them both with a letter outlining the problem and seeking their, and their constituents' participation, but also noting that the nature of participation had not been defined yet as it would be done in collaboration with the charities and patients and would partly depend on the numbers who wanted to become involved.

Seventy five charities responded, and these responses were followed up by two questionnaires. The first was used to elicit further details about the organisation and whether it represented/comprised any of the higher risk patient groups described above. The second questionnaire was provided to one of the group membership to gain information about personal experience with anticoagulants. Recipients to these questionnaires were asked to indicate a willingness to participate in a workshop.

Twenty two organisations and 45 patients responded, 18 of which expressed interest in the workshop.

Organisational responses:

- 19 (86%) declared membership which included the frail and those over 70 years
- Four (18%) had members whose first language is not English
- Three (14%) did not believe that sufficient and adequate information was provided to patients when they first commence anticoagulation therapy
- Four (18%) provided information to their membership about anticoagulants, two via meetings and two through supply of the *British Heart Foundation* booklet.

Patient responses:

- Age ranges of respondents
    Under 18 ($n=2$)
    18–0 ($n=11$)
    60–70 ($n=13$)
    over 70 ($n=19$).
- Ethnic origin:
    White ($n=39$),
    Asian ($n=1$),
    Black ($n=1$)
    Mixed race ($n=1$).

- Thirty eight people had been taking anticoagulants for more than one year, although five had taken them for less than a year, and one patient for less than four weeks
- Atrial fibrillation (26%) and heart valve replacement (23%) were the most common indications for use. One patient recorded that they did not know what they took anticoagulants for
- Treatment had commenced for the majority in hospital (91%), and all but one patient had been provided with information about

anticoagulants and the need for regular blood tests. However, three people (7%) did not understand the information they received

INR tests were conducted in the GP surgery (36%), at the hospital clinic (19%), other or multiple locations (18%), and one patient self-tested at home. INR results and necessary dose changes were communicated to the patients via a number of routes: hospital or surgery writing into the monitoring book; and phone call, letter or e-mail. Of these responders, only four did not hold a monitoring book. One further respondent self tested and recorded the result from their equipment, and one respondent stated that 'nobody tells me about my results or my dose'.

Patients taking warfarin were asked to record the tablet strengths they took (colours of each were described in the questionnaire), and also whether they had any problems in working out how many or which combination of tablets to take if their dose was changed. Eighteen held a single strength of warfarin, and 22 had combinations of two or three different strengths. One patient did not know what strength tablets they had. Six respondents stated that they had difficulty working out their dose and a further four had someone else complete this task for them.

Whilst the sample size for the warfarin group is small compared to the total number of patients receiving anticoagulation therapy, the responses to the questionnaires do reflect a level of commonality with the published literature on knowledge and numeric ability potentially affecting safe use of anticoagulant therapy. Key outcomes from patient participation are described in *Table 4.3*.

Table 4.3 . Key outcomes from patient participation

Process steps for anticoagulation therapy	Patient experience and barriers to safe use
Decision to treat	Wide range of experiences and involvement; use of medical jargon and abbreviations unhelpful. Lay knowledge of warfarin is as 'rat killer' and this use needs to be described in context of patient anticoagulation for some
Document and communicate diagnosis and treatment plan	Problems with information not communicated to patients' GPs. Poor communication with carers. Stroke patients receive less information and support than others. No planning for coping during first four weeks post-discharge, nor for longer-term regarding schooling, holidays, and other social events. Lack of information about effect of foods and alcohol on anticoagulation control. Overall discharge is the weakest yet critical stage
Arrange monitoring	Generally good although some do not understand INR. Lack of clarity about what the readings mean, especially when they vary between tests

Prescribe	Lack of communication between hospital consultant / clinic and GP when new drugs are introduced — other prescribers can be unaware of this. Conflicting information about aspirin; some are prescribed whilst others are told to avoid — the reasons for this need to be explained. Conflicting advice is a source of anxiety — patients do talk to one another and compare treatments
Prepare/dispense/supply	Some patients do not trust the system where they receive different packaging on each prescription supply. Whilst most are aware that warfarin tablets are colour coded, different manufacturers' packaging (primary and secondary) causes a degree of anxiety that they have received the correct medication At discharge it is vital that patients know to request further supplies before the 'to take home' supply runs out; reinforcing information and testing patients understanding
Administer dose	Use of 0.5mg warfarin tablets is not widespread, yet many patient and carers need to break 1mg tablets to produce the correct dose. Local policy of only using 3mg tablets and then prescribing 2mg daily dose causes very real problems for patients; local policies must be able to respond to patient need. Alternate day dosing regimes are difficult, especially for those with poor memories
Monitor treatment	Home testing, especially for children to avoid regular loss of school time, appreciated by patients but not by clinicians
Discontinue treatment	Dentists appear to be unaware of the specific needs of patients receiving anticoagulants and undertake treatment (from hygiene to multiple extractions) without managing the treatment or referring to others
Communication with patients/use of yellow book	The yellow book is an essential part of the process but GPs do not ask to see it There is a lack of good liaison between the NHS and schools, particularly around participation in sports, school trips, and likelihood of bruising The NHS should accept that patient groups form part of the pathway and can help patients when first diagnosed and throughout their anticoagulation therapy as a source of support

While *Table 4.3* illustrates that patient participation was useful in defining the problem and shaping the solutions, the benefits went far beyond research. For example, the evaluation of lay input showed that their awareness of the issues (benefits and risks) improved considerably as did staff awareness of the issues from the patient and carer perspective.

Shaping Corporate Products and Activities

While the above method is most efficient, where there is a clear target group who have experienced the condition or who have been identified as being at risk of harm, a different approach needs to be considered when dealing with more general subject areas. In this case the aim is to gather information and provide patient and public input into the forming of the NPSA's corporate role. In these kinds of projects such as developing the NPSA's Corporate and Business Plans or its mechanism to prioritise areas of work or its Research and Development Strategy, the NPSA invites people who have worked on other NPSA projects to participate and broadens this mix to include members of the public — usually recruited as members of Patient and Public Involvement Forums. Where this does not result in a broad enough spectrum of diversity the NPSA has used a range of other tactics for recruitment including advertising for participants.

Reporting PSIs to the NPSA

Prior to the NPSA's establishment there has been a Government commitment to ensure patients as well as others could report PSIs (DH, 2002). The NPSA knows of no other country with such a system. Thus from the NPSA's inception staff have worked with patients and others to identify the best way of capturing patient safety information from patients and the public (Williams and Hoey, 2002). One key consideration was a conceptual one of distinguishing between reporting for learning and reporting for accountability.

Historically, the Government and the NHS had established many systems and organisations dealing with accountability where patients can complain about NHS services or staff. For example patients can complaint to NHS Trusts, ICAS, The Healthcare Commission, The Health Ombudsman's Office, The General Medical Council (GMC), and the Nursing and Midwifery Council (NMC). However, none of these agencies were established to use the information to understand the nature of patient safety and to use the information on a system wide basis to reduce harm — this is the NPSA's remit (DH, 2001c). However much of the work the NPSA has completed with patients and patient groups suggest that unless we can show a direct benefit to the individual reporting the incident it will prove difficult to motivate patients to report to it (Williams and Hoey, 2002). This is why in part the role of the Patient Safety Observatory is important, because it will use third party data such as that gathered by ICAS and the Healthcare Commission for the purposes of patient safety rather than individual accountability.

Notwithstanding all of the above, patient reporting is an explicit Government policy commitment (DH, 2000c), and the NPSA has pressed ahead with developing patient reporting.

Patient and Public Reporting

The preferred method for patient reporting that was developed and tested combined a direct reporting e-Form completed on a computer and submitted electronically, with signposting to and from existing reporting services. This is available in multiple formats and also has the capacity to harvest data from third parties such as charities. A second key ingredient in the development of the reporting tool was the testing of the categories or datasets, whether the patient reports should use the same datasets as NHS staff or not, and to assess the implications for each option on the NPSA's ability to learn about the nature and volume of PSIs.

Early Learning

The NPSA undertook some early testing of incidents spontaneously reported by telephone, letter, e-mail and web enquiry during July 2001 and February 2005. These reports varied in length and detail but provided important insights into the types of errors or incidents that patients' and public have experienced. The data also provided an insight into the types of incidents patients' and the public perceive to be reportable. The main findings from this testing were:

- If patients were allowed to report in a totally unstructured way the NPSA would receive reports with a significant amount of missing information, including about how the reporter heard about the NPSA and year in which the incident occurred. Although this has not been a major issue for the NPSA the data could be a useful indicator of how successful other organisations are at signposting patients and the public to the NPSA's PPR system
- The majority of reports submitted occurred in England. This may reflect more awareness of PPR reporting in England or it may be an artefact of the proportion of patients treated in England versus Wales. No firm conclusions can be drawn at this stage
- Twenty-one percent of the patient safety incident reports contain information that there has been an inadequate response by the local healthcare team after the patient/carer has reported the incident to them
- Twenty three out of 170 PPR incidents were reported by healthcare staff rather than patients, family members or other groups that should report through PPR
- Three times as many incidents are reported indirectly to the NPSA, i.e. following a previous report being made to another organisation,

than directly to the NPSA (75 to 25 reports respectively)

- The incidents reported by patients are more likely to involve medication, access, admission, transfer, or discharge problems and consent, communication, confidentiality problems. These findings are consistent with other studies
(Change et al, 2005; Meredith et al, 2002)
- The free choice analysis identified some emerging sub-categories and examples which could be added to the listed examples from the current e-Form guidance.

It is clear that if the NPSA did not provide any structure for patients to reference their reports to it would not collect the information necessary for its purpose. However if it forced patients reporting into the Service's categorization it would also lose valuable data. Thus it has been necessary to develop a structured e-Form and dataset that is relevant and meaningful to patients and the public that complements the Service form in terms of information collected rather than mirror it.

Has Patient Involvement Made a Difference?

The benefits and disadvantages of the different methods of participation have been well documented (OPM, 2001). The NPSA finds that the methods it has developed work well because they allow for a deliberative, multipoint approach to participation, allow face-to-face interaction that provides a rich source of data, and they influence not only the NPSA products and services but is very culture (NPSA, 2004).

Levels of Participation

Moreover the levels of patient and/or public participation have changed over the lifespan of the NPSA with activities moving away from simple consultative events toward greater collaboration. However, it would be false to assume that the NPSA's activities were a true equal partnership since the NPSA is a Government agency and takes directions from the centre.

Examples of Participating at Different Levels

Collaborating with patients and members of the public

Participants have been involved throughout the processes of defining the problem, and developing solutions in regard of the following projects and work streams. They have collaborated with staff in a variety of ways on each issue and provided them with a high degree of collaborative control.

- Determining the processes the NPSA uses to prioritise its work
- Determining the actual priorities for action
- The method and tools used to enable patients and the public to report patient safety incidents directly to the NPSA
- The NPSA's stance and activities in regard of Being Open – a policy document aimed at motivating NHS staff to be more open with patients and families when things go wrong
- Identifying the problems and use of latex and non latex products in the care of latex sensitive patients
- Creating a safer environment on acute psychiatric wards
- Determining the patient safety priorities for people with learning disabilities
- Developing induction and support tools for patients and NPSA staff
- Identifying the safety issues concerned with the use of infusion devices and solutions to address them
- Reducing the risk of oral Methotrexate dosage error
- Actual patient and public reporting
- Training in Root Cause Analysis
- Defining and addressing the issues of anonymity and confidentiality of NPSA data
- Participating with the WHO International Alliance for Patient Safety
- Establishing an Advisory Board of service leaders in Wales
- Shaping the NPSA's focus, stance and activities.
- Determining the patient safety issues for some vulnerable groups of women
- Participating within the '*Clean Your Hands*' campaign
- Feeding into patients use of hip protectors to prevent fractured neck of femur in acute care setting
- Developing the NPSA's research and development strategy
- Developing the applicability of Seven Steps to Patient Safety with Patient Forums
- Understanding the contribution that supervised consumption can make in reducing accidental methadone overdose
- Developing staff training in the resuscitation of laryngectomy patients
- Reducing the risk of anaphylactic reactions in patients with known allergies

Consulting and informing patients and members of the public
Participants have been involved in shaping or choosing options within a fixed range and/

or have developed and shaped particular products such as the wording of guidance.

- Return advice information for parents/carers.
- Developing the NPSA's public and patient engagement campaign
- Developing a Patient Safety Assessment Framework
- Serious hazards of blood transfusion
- Wrong site surgery
- Safety tips for patients
- The NPSA has been collaborating with the Patient Safety Research Programme (PSRP) to issue a call for tenders on patients' involvement in their care as a way to improve patient safety
- Lay versions of the NPSA safety alerts such as on potassium, crash call numbers and nasal gastric tubes have been published

Conclusions

Has PPI Made a Difference? Impact of PPI on NPSA Staff

The most recent report suggests that patient and public involvement has had a big impact on staff in a variety of ways. It has provided an opportunity for patients and the public to review proposals and activities from a lay perspective and provides a 'reality check' for staff. In addition, it offers opportunities for NPSA staff to listen to its customers, it is an effective mechanism for receiving and responding to wider public input as distinguished from patients and carers, and it promotes improved relationships between patients, the public, and staff.

PPI also provides a vehicle for better communication between patients, the public, and staff; it provides a channel for information, needs, and concerns from patients to staff; it has helped the NPSA in planning to ensure that services focus on consumer needs and priorities; and it has actively helped the implantation of change. Furthermore, PPI has broadened some staff awareness for example the number of patients involved in the work of the NPSA listed above so far exceeds 500.

Whose Voices?

The figures below identify NPSA staff awareness of the profiles of people who have been involved in NPSA's work up to November 2004. *Table 4.4* identifies NPSA staff awareness of the profiles of people who have been involved in the NPSA's work up to November 2004, and represents the proportion and actual numbers against those staff who completed the questionnaire ($n=83$). This is heartening to see because it is important from the NPSA's point of view to work with people who make up the patient community, and highlights how the NPSA has been successful in working with a diversity of people.

Table 4.4: NPSA staff awareness

Category	Awareness levels of participation
Race	77 (93%) staff said they had involved people from Black and Asian ethnic minorities in their work
Religion	46 (55%) staff were aware of involving Muslims; 55 (66%) Christians; 45 (52%) Sikhs; 44 (53%) Hindus; 25 (30%) Buddhists; 42 (50%) atheists; and 47 (56%) Jews
Disability	57 (68%) staff said they had involved physically disabled people; 31 (37%) with people with sensory impairments; 43 (52%) with learning disabilities; and 44 (53%) with people with mental health problems
Sexuality	Staff were aware of involving 36 (43%) lesbians; 42 (50%) gay people, 26 (31%) bisexuals, and 19 (23%) trans-gender people
Geography	63 (76%) staff were aware of involving people from the north east; 61 (73%) from the north west; 61 (73%) from the east midlands; 59 (71%) from the west Midlands; 66 (80%) from the south east; 53 (64%) from South Wales; 54 (65%) from North Wales; and 53 (64%) from mid-Wales
Age	15 (18%) staff said they had involved children in their work and 28 (34%) said they had involved retired people
Literacy and language	35 (43%) staff were aware of involving people with low literacy levels and 51 (61%) whose first language is not English

Impact on Patients and the Public

Each piece of work usually has included an evaluation. Commonly patient feedback is very positive. Indeed just the fact that the NPSA is reaching out and is interested in their views with the intention of using them for a good purpose is welcomed. However over the three years the NPSA has worked with patients something else has taken place — a cultural shift with lay participation becoming embedded within the NPSA (NPSA, 2005b).

Impact on Safety

The recommendations following the Bristol inquiry have had far reaching consequences for patient and public participation in the operation of the NHS and in issues of patient safety. Patients, carers and others are actively involved in aspects of safety in NHS health care — as individual agents for their own health, and as participants in defining safety problems and patient safety solutions. However, many are astonished by the size and scope of NHS activity when exposed to it in any detail. Moreover their awareness of the level of PSI's taking place is very low. This means that the NPSA and all healthcare organisations dealing with patients need to plan carefully how to share issues of risk and use data and information consistently in order to empower patients to make informed decisions.

Moreover such organisations need to assess and meet the needs of patients and the public at both the individual and group level in order to provide equality of opportunity in decision making. They also need to consider the appropriate time to negotiate the level and nature of participation to ensure it is proportionate to the task and that it adds real value. The benefits can be great: within the NPSA it has influenced the focus, policies, plans, products and services of the NPSA; it has enabled learning, resources and expertise to be shared in ways that otherwise would not have taken place between different groups; and it has benefited all those who have been involved. Moreover the products developed and used nationally within England and Wales and the NPSA's commitment to patient participation has been recognised internationally by many organisations including the World Health Organisation's Alliance for Patient Safety.

Does the NHS Have a Memory?

The NHS is beginning to develop a framework to hold is memory. The development of the NPSA's National Reporting and Learning System (NRLS) alongside the application of tools such as Root Cause Analysis (RCA) all help capture, store, share and apply information that should result in fewer patients being harmed and patient reporting has had a key role to play in this area of learning. We hope to have demonstrated that patient safety cannot be achieved without patient participation and involvement. Patients often see things differently to the way staff see things. Patients may also interpret events and information differently from staff as a result of their individual experience and perspective. Such information is very useful to the NHS in understanding safety problems both from a scientific standpoint (e.g. a patient saw something clinicians did not see) and a subjective cultural one (e.g. patients may interpret risk differently from staff). Patients therefore report incidents differently compared to NHS staff. However the benefits of patient and lay participation generally go much further than providing new information — they change the processes and products of organisational development. The measures in assessing whether the range and levels of participation have been worthwhile will be determined in part by stakeholders' commitment to sustain an approach that is not easy and that sometimes can be intensely frustrating, but worthwhile for all concerned.

References

Barach P, Small SD (2000) Reporting and preventing medical mishaps: lessons from non-medical near miss reporting systems. *BMJ* **320**: 759–63

Chang A, Schyve PM, Croteau RJ, O'Leary DS, Loeb JM (2005) The JCAHO patient safety event taxonomy: a standardized terminology and classification schema for near misses and adverse events. *Int J Quality Health Care* **17**(2): 95-105

Coulter A (2002) *The autonomous patient: ending paternalism in medical care.* Nuffield Trust, London

Cousins D, Harris W (2003) Preventing patient safety incidents with anticoagulants. A scoping paper for NPSA Management Team. (February). NPSA, London

Cousins D, Harris W (in press) The risk assessment of anticoagulation therapy. NPSA, London

Cullen DJ, Bates DW, Small SD et al (1995) The incident reporting system does not detect adverse drug events: a problem for quality improvement. *J Comm J Qual Improv* **21**: 541-548

DH (1998) *A First Class Service: Quality in the new NHS.* Stationery Office, London

DH (2000a) *The NHS Plan: A Plan for Investment, A Plan for Reform.* Stationery Office, London

DH (2000b) *An Organisation with a Memory.* Stationery Office, London

DH (2001a) *Shifting the Balance of Power within the NHS: Securing Delivery.* Stationery Office, London

DH (2001b) *The Social Care Act 2001 (Section 11).* Stationery Office, London

DH (2001c) *Statutory Instrument 2001 No 1742 and 1743: Directions to the National Patient Safety Agency (July).* Stationery Office, London

DH (2002) *Learning from Bristol: The Department of Health's Response to the Report of the Public Inquiry into children's heart surgery at the Bristol Royal Infirmary 1984-1995.* Stationery Office, London

DH (2003a) *Making Amends. Clinical Negligence and Its Costs.* Stationery Office, London

DH (2003b) *NHS Complaints Reform: Making Things Right.* Stationery Office, London

DH (2004a) *Independent Complaints Advocacy Service. The First Year of ICAS.* Stationery Office, London

DH (2004b) *Chief Executives Report to the NHS (December).* Stationery Office, London

Florin D, Dixon J (2004) Public involvement in health care. *BMJ* **328**: 159-161

Institute for Safe Medication Practices (2003) *Safe Medicine: Protect Yourself From Medication Errors: premier issue.* ISMP, Huntington Valley

JCAHO (2002) Speak up: national campaign urges patients to join safety efforts (Press Release 14) (March)

Kennedy I (2001) *Learning from Bristol: The Report of the Public Inquiry into Children's Heart Surgery at the Bristol Royal Infirmary 1984-1995 Bristol Royal Infirmary Inquiry* (CM 5207). Stationery Office, London

Kingston MJ, Evans SM, Smith BJ, Berry JG (2001) Attitudes of doctors and nurses towards incident reporting: a qualitative analysis. *Med J Aust* **181**(1): 36-9

Lawton R, Parker D (2002) Barriers to incident reporting in a healthcare system. *Quality and Safety in Health Care* **11**: 15-18

Meredith AB, Makeham SM, Dovey M, Kidd MR (2002) An international taxonomy for errors in general practice: a pilot study. *Med J Aust* **177**(2):68-72

Modernisation Agency (2002) *Creating Effective and Continuous Involvement. The Improvement Leaders Guide.* NHS Modernisation Agency, London

National Consumer Council (2002) *Involving consumers – everyone benefits.* NCC, London

NPSA (2002) *Speaking Up Saves Lives: Engaging The Public in NPSA's Work. NPSA (June).* London. NPSA.

NPSA (2004) *Overview of Patient Involvement activities within NPSA's work. Report to the Board (December).* London. NPSA

NPSA (2005a) *Building a Memory: Preventing Harm, Reducing Risks and Improving Patient Safety. The National Reporting and Learning System and the Patient Safety Observatory Report.* London. NPSA

NPSA (2005b) *Overview of Patient Participation activities within NPSA's work: Report to the Board (November).* London. NPDA

Office Public Management (2001) *Signposts: A practical guide to public and patient involvement in Wales.* Cardiff. OPM

Vincent C, Coulter A (2002) Patient safety: what about the patient? *Quality and Safety in Health Care* **11**: 76-80

Vincent C et al (2001) PSIs in British Hospitals Preliminary Retrospective Record Review. *BMJ* **322**: 517-9

Waring JJ (2005) Beyond Blame: Cultural Barriers to Medical Incident Reporting. *Social Sciences and Medicine* **60**(9):1927-1935

Warnes, J (2003) *Extrapolating Vincent: A brief report on extending the results of the study by Vincent et al.* London. NPSA

Weingart SN, Ship AN, Aronson MD (2002) Confidential clinician reported surveillance of adverse events among medical inpatients. *J Gen Intern Med* **15**: 470–7

Williams S, Hoey A (2002) *Involving your consumers – what works? A report for the National Patient Safety Agency.* Consumerhealth Consulting (December)

CHAPTER 5

Staffing for Safety

Elizabeth West and Cherrill Scott

In the past, hospitals were often seen as dangerous places, where only the poor and isolated would seek refuge. In Britain, hospitals were transformed in the latter half of the 19th century by medical advances and by the development of the nursing profession (Black, 2005). These reforms transformed public perception of hospital care for many generations. However, public confidence in hospitals has recently been shaken. Department of Health (DH) surveys have repeatedly revealed that many NHS hospitals fall below acceptable standards of hygiene and the media has highlighted the dangers of hospital-acquired infection, malnourishment and the uncomfortable trolley waits that are sometimes associated with hospital care in the UK. While patients often give a positive overall evaluation of their hospital care, they can be highly critical of specific aspects of the physical, emotional and social care they have received.

Concerns about the fundamental aspects of patient safety in hospital were stimulated by the publication in the United States of the Institute of Medicine's report *'To Err is Human'* (Kohn et al, 1999), which suggested that many lives were lost each year as a result of medical errors, accidents and adverse events. Although a similar report has yet to be written about the UK, there are few reasons to suspect that the situation is very different here. The ramifications of the focus on safety in health care have been profound on both sides of the Atlantic. Increased funding was made available for research on patient safety, including research on the size and composition of the nursing workforce. Over the last few years, a number of important studies on the link between characteristics of the nursing workforce and patients outcomes have been published.

In this chapter we examine some of these key studies, assess the strengths and weaknesses of the evidence, and draw out some of the implications for policy and practice. Our main argument is that while there is some evidence that nurse staffing levels and the composition of the nursing workforce are linked to patient mortality and adverse events, the need for public debate, political action and further investment in research in this area remains profound.

What are the Consequences of Staffing Shortages?

The size of the nursing workforce and the ways in which the workforce is deployed has implications for the number of patients that each nurse is responsible for in the course of a shift and consequently for the amount of care that each patient receives. Although the current shortage of nurses is acknowledged in many countries, the consequences of the shortages in terms of quality and safety are seldom discussed. It is important therefore to connect the availability of nursing resources to qualitative aspects of patient's experiences in hospital.

Aiken et al (2001) reported that many nurses in the United States, Canada and Germany leave their work feeling that some essential nursing tasks have not been done. In all countries, nurses were performing housekeeping duties, transporting patients, and coordinating ancillary services while reporting that they did not have enough time for oral and skin care, comforting and teaching patients, or developing and updating care plans. Similar findings emerged from a survey of London nurses, which showed that many nursing tasks were being neglected in acute hospitals due to a lack of time, tools or training (West, Barron and Reeves 2005). Most of the respondents to this survey (64%) felt overworked, and many said they had insufficient time to provide nursing care, such as addressing patients' anxieties, fears and concerns, helping patients to the toilet, and answering call buttons. London nurses spent significant amounts of time searching for essential resources, such as linen or bathing aids.

The implications for quality and safety are obvious as is the potential impact that such experiences might have on the self-esteem and job satisfaction of nurses who are aware that they are unable to provide the levels of care to which they aspire (Reeves et al, 2005). There is clearly a need for hospitals to monitor how they are using trained staff and to institute measures to ensure that nurses are focused on providing nursing care rather than housekeeping and transport.

Evidence of a different kind about the implications of inadequate nurse staffing is contained in an official enquiry into a serious breach of safety that resulted in a patient's death following routine surgery (NHS Executive, 1999). Although the subsequent report acknowledged that there were many factors leading to an unsafe environment for clinical care, it was highly critical of nursing management for not establishing robust, regularly audited systems for setting nurse staffing levels. This led to a situation where there were low numbers of qualified nurses on the wards (often below the establishment agreed by the hospital), heavy reliance on bank and agency nurses, no clinical supervision, and lack of differentiation between the roles and clinical responsibilities of registered and non-registered nursing staff. The report also highlighted the importance of taking the ward design into account: in this case nurses could not see critically ill patients from the nursing station.

While surveys and case studies are useful sources of evidence, observational studies provide information about the relationship between nursing characteristics and patient outcomes on a larger scale. Studies of this kind try to determine the impact of nursing by controlling statistically for all the other sources of variation in patient outcomes and are intended to be generalisable to wider populations of hospitals and patients. The next section reviews some of the most important recent studies of this type.

Evidence of the Link between Staffing and Patient Safety: Recent Studies

In the USA, Linda Aiken has pioneered research on patient outcomes and has produced an impressive body of work on the impact of nursing (Aiken et al, 1994; Aiken et al, 1999). A recent study (Aiken et al, 2002) of Pennsylvania hospitals showed that after adjusting for patient and hospital characteristics, each additional patient per nurse increased both patient mortality and the likelihood of failure to rescue by about 7%. Additional patients also increased the likelihood of nurses experiencing burnout and job dissatisfaction. A later study using the same data showed that a 10% increase in the proportion of nurses holding a bachelor's degree was associated with a 5% decrease in patient mortality and the odds of failure to rescue. Therefore, in addition to the number of nurses, the educational composition of the workforce seems to be important.

A number of other studies support the link between characteristics of the nursing workforce and patient mortality. Tourangeau et al (2002) conducted a study of nurses in Ontario which showed that a richer skill mix and higher average number of years of experience of nurses on the unit both decreased mortality. The 'dose' of nursing was not found to be related to 30 day mortality.

Another Canadian study conducted by Estabrookes et al (2005) used multi-level modelling to show that higher nurse education levels, a richer nurse skill mix and better nurse-physician relationships reduced mortality rates, while a higher proportion of casual or temporary positions was associated with higher mortality rates. A recent study of over 100,000 patients in the US found that higher levels of staffing by registered nurses (RNs) was associated with lower levels of mortality. However the opposite was true of Licensed Practice Nurses (LPNs), where higher levels were associated with higher mortality (Person et al 2004). Even after extensive adjustment, higher levels of staffing by registered nurses were associated with lower levels of in-hospital mortality.

A study of staffing characteristics that has been the subject of a great deal of media attention was conducted by Needleman et al (2002). This study is particularly interesting because of its size (over five million medical and one million surgical patients), and because it examined mortality, failure to rescue and adverse events. They found that higher number of hours of care provided by registered nurses to medical patients was associated with a shorter length of stay and lower rates of some adverse events (urinary tract infections [UTI], upper gastro-intestinal [GI] bleeding, pneumonia, shock or cardiac arrest, and failure to rescue). The number of hours of care provided by registered nurses to surgical patients was associated with lower rates of UTI and failure to rescue — defined as death from pneumonia, shock, cardiac arrest, upper GI bleeding, sepsis or deep venous thrombosis — but they found no association between increased numbers of registered nurses and death in hospital, once failure to rescue patients had been accounted for. Nor did they find a relationship between the number of other health care workers providing nursing care, such as nurses' aides, and the occurrence of adverse events. Their main finding was that a higher proportion of care provided by registered nurses as well as a greater number of hours of care provided by registered nurses lowered the rate of adverse events, some of which were then linked to mortality.

Another recent study provides some weak evidence of the impact of staffing levels on adverse events. Kovner et al (2002) found that higher registered nursing staffing levels had negative associations with four adverse events, but these estimates were statistically significant ($p<0.05$) only for pneumonia.

Stronger evidence comes from another study conducted in Pennsylvania. Unruh (2003) used data from all the acute hospitals in the state from 1991 to 1997 to study the link between registered nurses and a number of adverse events: lung collapse, pressure sores, falls, pneumonia, post-treatment infections and UTIs. The main findings were that hospitals that had fewer registered nurses had higher rates of nearly all adverse events, and hospitals that had a lower proportion of licensed nurses had a greater incidence of decubitus ulcers and pneumonia. This study is particularly interesting because it used data gathered over time, which strengthens the researchers ability to make causal claims about the links between the independent and the dependent variables.

Research in this tradition has sometimes been criticised for its lack of attention to theory, and for a failure to draw on organisational sociology where there is a long tradition of investigating organisational performance. In contrast, Mark et al (2003) tested hypotheses drawn from contingency theory about how characteristics of the hospital (complexity of services, teaching status, volatility in the pattern of admissions and number of beds) and unit (level of experience, education and skill mix of nurses in the unit, size, availability of support services and the complexity of patient care provided) impacts on professional nursing practice and in turn how this affects nurse and patient outcomes, including satisfaction, medication errors and falls. Professional nursing practice appeared to be lower in large units and those that experienced high volatility in admissions, and higher in units providing highly technical services and where services were available to support nurses. At both hospital and unit level professional nursing practice had a strong positive effect on nurses' work satisfaction and was associated with lower turnover rates. It had, however, no discernible impact in this study on any other patient or nurse outcomes.

A later study (Mark et al, 2004) investigated the relationship between nurse staffing levels and quality of care in a sample of US hospitals. The authors argue that by using a 'dynamic panel model' they can evaluate the effects of change in nurse staffing on change in quality of care, which again strengthens their ability to make causal claims. Estimates were obtained using the method of 'first differences'. Key outcome measures were mortality, pneumonia, decubitis and UTI. A risk-adjusted estimated probability of death was generated for each patient, which was used to calculate the annual expected number of deaths and complication rates for each hospital. The key claim made in the paper is that there is a non-linear relationship between registered nurse staffing and mortality. Mortality fell until registered nurse staffing reached 4.62 full time equivalents (FTEs) per 1,000 inpatient days. There were no clear associations between nurse staffing and the other three quality measures.

McGillis Hall et al (2003) investigated how the proportion of regulated nursing staff and skill mix (defined as the mix of RNs/RPNs and unregulated workers) affected patients' functional status, medical status, experience of pain and perceptions of nursing care. They found that the proportion of regulated staff was associated with better functioning at discharge. When the skill mix included RNs and unregulated workers (rather than RNs/RPNs and UWs), patients had better pain outcomes at discharge. Obstetric patients were more satisfied with their care in settings that had a higher proportion of regulated staff.

A later study by McGillis Hall et al (2004) investigated the effects of the same nursing characteristics on adverse events (falls, medication errors, wound infections and urinary tract infections) and on healthcare costs. Medication errors and wound infections were higher in units that employed fewer professional nursing staff and the latter were related to length of nurses' experience. In settings that included a lower proportion of professional nursing staff, more nursing hours were used. This may be because the patients had more complex nursing needs.

This brief review of some recent studies shows that the evidence of a link between staffing characteristics and mortality and adverse events has accumulated rapidly over the last few years. There are signs of theoretical and methodological developments that may anticipate further work that can deliver even stronger and more compelling evidence. The foundations of this literature on the impact of nursing have been laid by recent work in North America, facilitated undoubtedly by numerous factors including high levels of concern about patient safety, funding for large scale studies, and the availability of high quality administrative data. In the next section we turn our attention to related studies that have been conducted in the UK, where the culture of research and health care generally differs markedly in a number of respects.

Evidence on Staffing and Safety: UK Studies

There are far fewer studies of nurse staffing in the UK that could compare with the analyses of the large data sets on staffing and outcomes discussed above. Carr-Hill et al (1992) conducted a ward-based investigation to test whether the effectiveness of nursing care was affected by different nursing skill mixes, and by different ways of organising nursing care (for example, team allocation or primary nursing). They observed care in seven medical and eight surgical wards, and used the Qualpacs package to assess the quality of nursing care. An outcome measurement tool was developed which identified eight specific areas over which ward nurses have major control. Three of these areas, arguably, are directly related to patients' safe recovery after treatment:

- Patient nutrition and hydration
- Pressure sores/skin integrity
- Intravenous therapy.

The researchers found that better overall quality of care was provided by higher grades of nursing staff, but that standards could be maintained if higher grades worked alongside lower grades. They concluded that investment in qualified staff, post-registration education and the systematic organisation of nursing care paid dividends in the delivery of good quality patient care. They also commented on the difficulty of conducting research in this area, given the many variables affecting patient outcomes. This study could not provide the sort of information required for setting specific nurse:patient ratios or for developing a universal management tool that could be used to monitor changes in staffing and skill mix.

Other commentators drew attention to the continuing lack of sufficiently robust research evidence to inform management decisions on staffing (McKenna, 1995; Meyer and Spilsbury, 1998).

Jarman et al (1999) analysed English data to investigate the link between doctor numbers and mortality, but also reported a correlation between increased mortality and higher numbers of non-registered 'A' grade staff, but none with the measure of 'total nurses per bed'. However, the quality of the nursing data they used is thrown into doubt by the findings of two recent investigations which analysed data on nurse staffing and outcomes from 6,000 wards in England and Wales (Audit Commission, 2001; Healthcare Commission, 2005). The 2001 study was limited by the poor quality of routine data, and the authors were unable to draw any conclusions about the impact of differing nursing numbers and skill mixes on selected patient outcomes (the reported incidence of pressure ulcers, patient accidents, and patient complaints).

The 2005 study reported an improvement in the type and quality of data provided by NHS hospital trusts. Data were collected at ward level on accidents and incidents, drug errors and needlestick injuries. It was found that the higher the proportion of registered nurses, the lower the number of accidents and incidents, and the lower the incidence of pressure ulcers. One apparently conflicting finding was that trusts with a higher proportion of registered nurses reported more drug errors. The report suggests that this may reflect a relationship between wards where more drugs are given, and wards with more registered nurses. (It may also reflect that some hospitals have a better 'safety culture' and have robust systems for reporting errors).

Whilst this study provides further evidence of a positive association between registered nurse input and improved outcomes, the authors state that it will be difficult to draw firm conclusions until data quality is improved further, and until the development of outcome measures that are shown to be sensitive to nursing. Research on the link between nursing characteristics and patient outcomes in the UK will be limited until further investment is made in the collection of high quality patient data sets.

Assessing the Evidence

The recent growth in large scale studies linking nursing characteristics to patient outcomes has prompted many to ask what scientific inferences can be drawn from the current evidence base. A number of large, systematic reviews of research of the evidence of the impact of nurse patient ratios and the composition of the nursing workforce in terms of education and experience on patient outcomes have recently been published (US Agency for Healthcare Research and Quality, 2003; Carr-Hill et al, 2004; and Hewitt et al, 2004). The most recent systematic review, by Lankshear et al (2005a), identified 22 studies conducted in acute settings since 1990. To be included in this review studies had to have adjusted for patient and hospital characteristics and had to have been conducted in more than one unit. The majority of the research was cross-sectional and used data from large public administrative data sets.

The authors identified nine large acute studies found a significant inverse relationship between registered nurse staffing levels and mortality rates (Aiken et al 1994; Silber et al 1995; Silber et al 2000; Aiken et al 2002; Tourangeau et al 2002; Mark et al, 2004; Person et al 2004), and four studies that found a negative association between nurse staffing and failure to rescue (Silber et al, 1995; Silber et al, 2000; Aiken et al, 2002; Needleman et al, 2002). They conclude that although there is a great deal of variability in the quality of the studies, there is a consistent pattern of results, particularly with regard to mortality. However the pattern of associations between characteristics of the nursing workforce and complications was described as 'less consistent', with a number of studies showing a relationship to pneumonia (seven of eight studies), urinary tract infections (six studies), decubitus ulcers (four studies), falls (four studies) and wound infections (two studies). Again, the authors caution against interpreting existing research as providing evidence for a causal relationship between nursing workforce characteristics and patient outcomes, mainly because the majority of studies are cross-sectional. Staffing levels may be indicative of other features of a 'good hospital' and if this is the case simply altering the number of nurses would not itself improve patient safety. The authors also suggest a curvilinear relationship, which would imply that there are limits to using qualified nurse staffing levels as a tool for improving the quality of care.

Implications for Policy and Practice

In response to the emerging evidence base and in reaction to what were perceived as cost-cutting reductions in registered nurse numbers by employers, some professional nursing associations have lobbied energetically for mandatory, minimum staffing ratios for qualified staff. So far, there have been two examples of successful lobbying: the states of California, USA; and Victoria, Australia, where the respective legislatures have laid down compulsory nurse:patient ratios for different clinical areas, in different categories of hospital. In California, for example, legislation in 1999 required universal adoption on medical and surgical wards of a 6:1 ratio, giving 4 registered nursing hours per patient. It had been planned to increase this to 5:1 (giving 4.8 registered nursing hours) in January 2005, but this move was postponed after state regulators found that more than half the hospitals they reviewed were in breach of the 1999 ratios. According to the American Nurses Association (ANA) four other states in the USA have now introduced legislation that requires specific nurse:patient ratios in certain units, such as paediatric intensive care (ANA, 2004). The process of reaching agreement on these mandatory ratios in California and Victoria was difficult and protracted: one of the main areas of disagreement between the negotiating bodies representing employers and nurses focused on the choice of method for assessing workload and measuring patient dependency, both of which are key factors in determining staffing ratios.

Apart from the political fights involved and the difficulties of monitoring implementation, there are other objections to a mandatory approach, such as its inflexibility and the difficulties of calibrating ratios that will ensure 'safety'

(Scott, 2003; Buchan, 2004). The ANA has chosen to support an approach that does not set specific, mandatory ratios: the Quality Nursing Care Act of 2005 (Safe Staffing Systems). This measure is aimed at preventing employers from stretching nursing staff with unsafe patient loads, from enforcing overtime working and directing nurses to work on units without prior training and orientation. The Act would establish a requirement for minimum staffing ratios, but rather than setting a specific numeric ratio, it requires the establishment of a staffing system that 'ensures a number of registered nurses on each shift …to provide for appropriate staffing levels for patient care'. The criteria for establishing a staffing system include:

- Input from direct-care registered nurses
- Basis in the numbers and acuity levels of patients and the number of admissions and discharges on each shift
- Reflect staffing levels recommended by specialty nursing organisations public reporting of the daily numbers of qualified and unqualified staff on each shift
- Whistle-blower protection for registered nurses and others who may have concerns about staffing (ANA, 2005).

There are significant differences between the situation of registered nurses in the USA and the UK. Shuldham (2004) notes that in the USA, if more nurses are rostered than are needed for the number of patients or the acuity of the ward, some staff may be sent home without pay.

Nevertheless, concerns about the impact of a possible dilution of nursing skill mix on quality and safety are generating debate around the issue of mandatory ratios in the UK Royal College of Nursing (Scott, 2003). The RCN in Scotland is lobbying for a legal requirement to be placed on NHS Boards to ensure appropriate staffing levels, which would be determined locally and may include nurse:patient ratios. Since the 1970s, central government in the UK has avoided giving top-down guidance about staffing levels, on the grounds that this is a matter for local management in the NHS (and thereby, presumably, contributing to the wide variation in staffing levels and costs reported by the Audit Commission and the Healthcare Commission). There are some existing guidelines on staffing in specialist areas, such as adult and paediatric patient care and mental health wards; these have been developed by expert groups, and it is considered good practice for managers to refer to these when making decisions about staffing levels in nursing and other professions. The trend in workforce planning is increasingly towards using multi-disciplinary as opposed to uni-disciplinary approaches (Shuldham, 2004).

It seems clear from events in California (USA) and Victoria (Australia) that decisions about mandatory nurse:patient ratios are likely to be contested between employers and professional nurses, with the latter group asserting the importance of professional judgment grounded in experience. As we have seen, most of the recent, high quality research studies do not provide a guide as to exactly how many nurses are required in different settings to provide safe care to patients with different needs. Lang et al (2004) systematically reviewed studies of the effects of nurse staffing on patient, nurse employee, and hospital outcomes published between 1980 and 2003 to determine whether they could guide the setting of minimum nurse-patient ratios in acute care hospitals. They concluded that while the evidence suggests that higher levels of nurse staffing is associated with lower failure-to-rescue rates, lower inpatient mortality rates, and shorter hospital stays, the literature offers no support for specific, minimum nurse:patient ratios for acute care hospitals, especially in the absence of any adjustments for skill and the characteristics of patients (risk adjustment). There is, as yet, no firm evidence on the longer-term effectiveness of the nurse:patient ratios in California and Victoria (Buchan, 2004).

In the absence of universally-applicable formulae for staffing levels and skill mix, what other practical support is available to managers of nursing who have to make such crucial decisions? Good management practice requires a systematic and business-like approach to workforce planning. However, the use of management information tools to help determine staffing requirements has not been widely adopted in the UK, despite persistent official encouragement (Audit Commission, 1992; NHS Executive, 1995). Resistance has been partly due to the nursing time involved in collecting data, but more to the professional view that decisions about ward establishments should not be informed by standardised workload measurement tools which do not take sufficient account of the complexity of the situation at ward level (Scott, 2003).

On an operational basis, managers have to take account of the skills of available staff, the supervision required by the less skilled staff, the levels of patient dependency (which may fluctuate unpredictably), the incidence of emergency admissions, and ward layout (Shuldham, 2004). Indeed, the International Council of Nurses advised that there was no such thing as an 'optimum skill mix', and the process of deciding on skill mix should be an 'on-going and creative process' (ICN, 1994).

Research has shown that the professional judgment of experienced nurses about staffing requirements can produce comparable results to more 'objective' management tools (Taket et al, 1983) — a reassuring finding given that there is inevitably an element of subjective judgment involved in using such tools. Other research suggests the need for a system of checks and balances in any system that relies primarily on professional judgment. Procter (1992) found that there were subtle ways in which organisational constraints could distort professional judgment over time. Ward sisters might become accustomed to working with in-house staffing levels that were below the agreed establishments, and plan rotas on the basis of self-imposed 'norms' about minimum staffing levels. Agency or bank staff were commonly used to keep staffing levels up to these (low) levels, rather than being used to compensate for unforeseen shortfalls in the establishment due, for example, to staff sickness. Procter's findings anticipate the breaches of patient safety associated with weak nursing management reported a few years later at a hospital in England (NHS Executive, 1999).

In summary, perhaps the best that can be said at the moment is that determining safe staffing levels is an important aspect of clinical judgment and managerial decision-making that should be guided by relevant expert recommendations and an understanding of the existing research evidence, which although unable at the moment to give exact figures, seems to favour staffing acute wards with more rather than less nurses, and trying to recruit and retain a nursing workforce that is highly educated and experienced.

Nursing establishments, however decided upon initially, should be regularly reviewed to allow for changes in the patient population and professional practice. Ideally, management information on outcomes relating to quality and safety should be used in conjunction with detailed data on ward staffing, to monitor the situation.

Even though we do not have enough evidence to devise an evidence-based policy that includes exact numbers, the consequences of inadequate staffing are so grave that we must err on the side of caution and implement safe staffing policies now. This should include looking at findings of studies that relate not just to ratios and skill mix, but to the organisation and management of the nursing workforce. For example, Kay (2005) cites research which suggests that the risk of making an error increased significantly when a nurse worked shifts longer than 12 hours, worked significant overtime, or worked more than 40 hours per week.

Implications for Budgets

It is estimated that in the UK, adverse events affect 10% of admissions to hospital and cost the NHS an estimated £2 billion (Lankshear et al, 2005b). Medication errors are believed to account for one quarter of all adverse incidents; and in the USA 38% of medication errors are believed to be attributable to nurses (Leape, 2002).

The costs to the NHS of hospital-acquired infection and pressure ulcers are high; again, these are outcomes which have been found attributable to nurse staffing levels. This suggests that investing money in adequate nurse staffing can be offset against the potential financial gains from shorter lengths of stay and reduced treatment.

There is some evidence to support this (Sovie and Jawad, 2001; McCue et al, 2003), and recent work by a group of economists (Rothberg et al, 2005) provides further evidence. They conducted a cost-effectiveness analysis comparing patient-to-nurse ratios ranging from 8:1 to 4:1. Patient mortality and length of stay data for different ratios were based on 2 large hospital level studies (Aiken et al, 2002; Aiken, 2003). They found that eight patients per nurse was the least expensive ratio but was associated with the highest patient mortality. Decreasing the number of patients per nurse improved mortality but increased costs steadily as the ratio declined from 8:1 to 4:1. The model was most sensitive to the effects of patient-to-nurse ratios on mortality. Lower ratios were most cost-effective when lower ratios shortened length of stay, and hourly wages were low. Across the entire range of these variables the cost of saving a life never exceeded US dollars $449,000, which is a much cheaper way of saving a life than many other interventions, for example screening which tends to be very expensive. These authors conclude that:

'...as a patient safety intervention, patient-to-nurse ratios of 4:1 are reasonably cost-effective and in the range of other commonly accepted interventions.'
Rothberg et al, 2005

Two recent UK studies focus on the relative costs and benefits of different approaches to nursing skill mix. The Audit Commission (2001) compared staff numbers (including qualified nurses, health care assistants and nursing auxiliaries) and average costs per bed across comparable wards and departments in similar types of hospital. It found significant variation in spending between different regions of the country, with particularly high staffing costs in NHS trusts with teaching hospitals, and in London hospitals. An analysis of relative costs per staff member showed that high-spending trusts employed more staff per bed, rather than more expensive (and presumably more highly-qualified) nurses. Unfortunately, due to the limitations of poor quality data, the report was unable to say anything conclusive about the links between nurse staffing costs and the quality of nursing care.

A repeat investigation was undertaken by the new Healthcare Commission which was able to draw on additional data from two national surveys, one of NHS staff and the other of patients (Healthcare Commission, 2005). Again, wide variation was found in the amounts spent on staffing between similar wards in different hospitals, and sometimes within the same hospital. Overall, staffing costs were determined by the total numbers of nurses employed, rather than the number of Whole Time Equivalent registered nurses (the unit used by the report as a measure of skill mix). The report concludes that spending more per staff member — that is, having a richer skill mix — is likely to improve the safety and quality of care, as well as raising patients' satisfaction with care. There is a caveat: some trusts were found to produce good results with a relatively lean skill mix, and the authors state that it is important to understand how this is achieved.

These early attempts to draw out the economic implications about decisions about nurse staffing show how high quality primary research can be used to provide guidance to clinicians, managers and policy makers in a common language — the language of finance — that can be understood across professional boundaries. However, the predictive ability and usefulness of the economic calculations depends heavily on the quality of the original estimates.

Conclusion

There is widespread concern about the safety of hospital care in many industrialized countries and healthcare organizations have been challenged to develop a new, more open attitude to discussing accidents and near misses and to examine the systemic causes of errors (West, 2001). At the same time, the current shortage of nurses is expected to increase as a significant proportion of the nursing workforce reaches retirement age, just as the demand for health care is expected to increase.

The discrepancies between supply and demand for nursing care render research into the link between characteristics of the nursing workforce and patient outcomes very important to policy and practice. We need to know much more, not just about how many nurses are needed to ensure patient safety, but also about how to deploy this scarce resource so that further investment in nursing is used cost-effectively.

We conclude that the emerging evidence base is impressive and compelling, not because of the features of any one study, but because of the consistency of the results across studies conducted in diverse locations. The relationship between characteristics of the nursing workforce (size, level of education and experience) and patient mortality is particularly convincing. If we are going to conduct studies of a similar kind in the UK we need more systematic efforts to collect high quality, risk adjusted data about patients' experiences and outcomes that can be compared across organizations, as well as much more detailed information about the nursing care that they received. Data of this kind can only be collected by those closely involved in care and it will take the energy, initiative, collaboration and collective action of clinicians, nurses and researchers to develop and disseminate an effective system. At the same time, we need to ensure that the next generation of nurse researchers has the skills in organizational theorizing and quantitative analysis to use the data, as well as a deep understanding of the political context within which research is interpreted and used. The need for building the research infrastructure that underpins patient safety remains profound.

References

AHRQ (2004) *Hospital Nurse staffing and Quality of Care Research in Action.* AHRQ, London

Aiken LH, Smith HL, Lake ET (1994) Lower Medicare mortality among a set of hospitals known for good nursing care. *Med Care* **32**: 771-87

Aiken LH, Sloane DM, Lake ET, Sochalski J, Weber AL (1999) Organization and outcomes of inpatient AIDS care. *Med Care* **37**: 760-72

Aiken LH, Clarke SP, Sloane D et al (2001) Nurses' reports on hospital care in five countries. *Health Affairs* **20**(3): 43-51

Aiken LH et al (2002) Hospital nurse staffing and patient mortality, nurse burnout, and job dissatisfaction *JAMA* **288**(16): 1987-93

Aiken LH et al (2003) Educational levels of hospital nurses and surgical patient mortality. *JAMA* **290**(12): 1617-23

ANA (2004) *2004 legislation: Staffing Plans and Ratios.* http://www.nursingworld. org/gova/state/2004/staffing.htm. (Accessed: 24 October 2005)

ANA (2005) *ANA Government Affairs.* http://vocusgr.vocus.com/grconvert1/webpub/ ana/ProfileBill.asp?BillID=6270&XSL. (Accessed 24 October 2005)

Audit Commission (1992) *Caring Systems: A Handbook for Managers of Nursing and Project Managers.* Her Majesty's Stationery Office, London

Audit Commission Acute Hospital Portfolio (2001) *Ward Staffing.* Audit Commission, London

Black N (2005) Rise and demise of the hospital: a reappraisal of nursing. *BMJ* **331**: 1394-1396

Buchan J (2004) *A Certain Ratio? Minimum Staffing Ratios in Nursing.* Royal College of Nursing, London

Carr-Hill R, Dixon P, Gibbs IK et al (1992) *Skill Mix and the Effectiveness of Nursing Care.* Centre for Health Economics, London

Carr-Hill R, Currie L, Dixon P (2004) *Skill Mix in Secondary Care: SDO Scoping Exercise. Final Report.* University of York Centre for Health Economics

Estabrooks CA, Midodzi WK, Cummings GG et al (2005) The impact of hospital nursing characteristics on 30 day mortality. *Nurs Res* **54**(2):74-84

Healthcare Commission (2005) *Ward Staffing London.* Commission for Healthcare Audit and Inspection, London

Hewitt C et al (2004) *Health Service Workforce and Health Outcomes — A Scoping Study.* NCCSDO, London

ICN (1994) *Planning Human Resources for Nursing.* ICN, Geneva: p 27

Jarman B, Gault S, Alves B et al (1999) Explaining differences in English hospital death rates using routinely collected data. *BMJ* **318**:1515-1520

Kay M (2005) A Brave New World: Imagining error-free health care. *AJN* **105**(3): 81–83

Kovner C, Jones C, Zhan C et al (2002) Nurse staffing and post-surgical adverse events: An analysis of administrative data from a sample of US hospitals: 1990–1996. *HSR* **37**: 611-629

Kohn LT, Corrigan JM, Donaldson MS (1999) *To Err is Human: Building a Safer Health Care System*. National Academy of Sciences, Washington DC

Lang TA et al (2004) Nurse-patient ratios: A systematic review of the effects of nurse staffing on patient, nurse employee, and hospital outcomes. *J Nurs Admin* **34**(7/8): 326-337

Lankshear A, Sheldon TA, Maynard A (2005a) Nurse staffing and healthcare outcomes: a systematic review of the international research evidence. *Adv Nurs Sci* **28**(2): 163-174

Lankshear A, Sheldon T, Maynard A, Smith K (2005b) *Health Policy Matters*: *Issue 10, July 2005*. Department of Health Sciences, University of York

Leape LL (2002) Reporting of adverse events. *N Engl J Med* **347**(20): 1633-1638

Mark BA et al (2003) Professional nursing practice: impact on organisational and patient outcomes. *J Nurs Admin* **33**(4): 224-34

Mark BA et al (2004) A longitudinal examination of hospital registered nurse staffing and quality of care. *Health Services Research* **39**(2): 279-300

McCue M, Mark BA, Harless DW (2003) Nurse staffing, quality and financial performance. *J Health Care Finance* **29**(4): 54-76

McGillis Hall L (2003) Nurse staffing models as predictors of patient outcomes. *Medical Care* **41**(9): 1096-109

McGillis Hall L et al (2004) Nurse staffing models, nursing hours, and patient safety outcomes. *J Nurs Admin* **34**(1): 41-5

McKenna HP (1995) Nursing skill mix substitutions and the quality of care: an exploration of assumptions from the research literature. *J Adv Nurs* **21**(3): 425–459

Meyer J, Spilsbury K (1998) *Defining the Nursing Contribution*. St Bartholomew School of Nursing and Midwifery, City University, London

Needleman J et al (2002) Nurse staffing levels and the quality of care in hospitals. *N Engl J Med* **346**(22): 1715-22

NHS Executive (1995) *Benefits Realisation Monograph on Nursing Information Systems London*. Department of Health, London

NHS Executive (1999) *The Review of Nursing at Eastbourne Hospitals NHS Trust*. Department of Health, London

Person SD et al (2004) Nurse staffing and mortality for medicare patients with acute myocardial infarction. *Med Care* **42**(1): 4-12

Procter S (1992) Subjectivity and objectivity in the measurement of nursing workload. *J Clin Nurs* **1**: 123-129

Rothberg MB, Abraham I, Lindenauer PK, Rose D (2005) Improving nurse-to-patient staffing ratios as a cost-effective safety intervention. *Medical Care* **43**(8): 785–791

Reeves R, West E, Barron D (2005) The impact of barriers to care on nurses' intentions to leave London hospitals. *Journal of Health Services Research and Policy* **10**(1): 5-9

Scott C (2003) *Setting Safe Staffing Levels*. Royal College of Nursing Institute, London

Shuldham C (2004) Nurse workforce planning in the UK: policies and impact. *J Nurs Manage* **12**(6): 388-392

Silber JH, Rosenbaum P, Ross R (1995) Comparing the contributions of groups of predictors: which outcomes vary with hospital rather than patient characteristics. *JASA* **90**: 7-18

Silber JH, Kennedy SK, Even-Soshan O et al (2000) Anesthesiologist direction and patient outcomes. *Anesthesiology* **93**: 152–163

Sovie MD, Jawad AF (2001) Hospital restructuring and its impact on outcomes: nursing staff regulations are premature. *J Nurs Admin* **31**(12): 588-600

Taket A, Beardsworth J, Rushworth V (1983) *Nurse Manpower Project for the NHS Management Inquiry: A comparison of some methods of estimating the requirements of nursing staff*. Department of Health and Social Security, London

Tourangeau AE et al (2002) Nursing related determinants of 30-day mortality for hospitalised patients. Canadian *J Nurs Res* **33**(4): 71-88

Unruh L (2003) Licensed nurse staffing and adverse events in hospitals. *Medical Care* **41**(1): 142-52

West E (2001) Organisational sources of safety and danger: Sociological contributions to the study of adverse events. *Quality in Health Care* **9**: 120–126

West E, Rafferty AM, Lankshear A (2004) *The Future Nurse: Evidence of the Impact of Registered Nurses on Patient Outcomes*. Royal College of Nursing, London

West E, Barron DN, Reeves R (2005) Overcoming the barriers to patient centred care: Time, tools and training. *J Clin Nurs* **14**(4): 435–43

CHAPTER 6

Improving Patient Safety Through Effective Risk Management

Philomena Fox

'Human beings make mistakes because the systems, tasks and processes they work in are poorly designed'
Professor Lucian Leape, Harvard School of Public Health

Every day over one million people are treated safely and successfully in the National Health Service (NHS). However, the Department of Health (DH, 2000) estimates that 1 in 10 patients admitted to NHS hospitals suffer unintentional harm, half of which are judged to have been preventable. As described in Chapter 1, there are conflicting accounts of the true level of patient safety incidents, which reinforces the fundamental importance of ensuring that we focus on the effective management of clinical risk. Effective risk management presents major challenges for organisations given the increasing complexity of healthcare coupled with the requirement to juggle competing and often conflicting priorities.

Organisational culture also impacts on how staff view patient safety. They may embrace it and feel secure in reporting mistakes and risks or they may feel frightened, threatened and isolated by the way they are treated (Firth-Cozens, 2001). The establishment of a patient safety culture that is just, fair and accountable is fundamental to an organisation's successful implementation of effective risk management.

This chapter highlights some of the national imperatives driving the patient safety agenda, provides a brief overview on the strategy used to manage risk across one organisation and presents a case study based on actual events.

National Imperatives

National Clinical Risk Management Standards
The NHS Litigation Authority (NHSLA) administers the Clinical Negligence Scheme for Trusts (CNST), which promotes effective management of clinical risk and provides a means for NHS organisations to fund the cost of clinical

negligence claims (NHSLA, 2005).

When an organisation joins the scheme it is assessed against a set of national standards. These standards are assessed progressively at three levels, and once organisations become compliant at one level they may apply for assessment at the next level. The general standards for acute NHS organisations cover a variety of risk areas, including consent, record keeping, incident reporting, medicines management, induction, training and assessment of competence. In addition to the general standards for acute NHS organisations, separate standards exist for Maternity Services.

Compliance at Level 1 of CNST demonstrates a structured approach to clinical risk management, whilst the higher level assessments concentrate on measuring how well this is integrated into everyday practice. The process offers a useful framework for organisations to develop and progress the patient safety agenda. Assessment by external assessors provides a valuable source of independent assurance, whilst highlighting good practice and identifying areas for improvement. In addition there is a financial incentive with discounts applied to the annual contribution an organisation pays to the scheme according to the level of compliance achieved.

The introduction of the CNST standards provided the incentive for NHS organisations to improve their risk management processes, and CNST accreditation is now well established across the NHS.

Although the standards have been specifically clinical in nature, in an effort to reduce the burden of healthcare inspection, work is underway to introduce a single set of integrated risk management standards for each type of organisation. These standards will incorporate organisational, clinical and health and safety risks and formal assessments are expected to commence in 2007. Further information on CNST can be found at www.nhsla.com.

The National Patient Safety Agency

The National Patient Safety Agency (NPSA) describes integrated risk management as the process of identification, assessment, analysis and management of all risks and incidents for every level of an organisation, and aggregation of the results at a corporate level (NPSA, 2004). In explaining the benefits of such an approach for local NHS organisations, the NPSA includes improved decision making, consistency, more effective planning and sharing learning across all areas of risk.

The publication *Seven Steps to Patient Safety* (NPSA, 2004) is a useful reference guide that provides organisations with a practical checklist against which to measure their performance and make improvements in patient safety. Examples of best practice are identified from across the country and a variety of tools to enhance patient safety are described. The *Seven Steps to Patient Safety* have been identified as:

- Step 1: Building a safety culture
- Step 2: Leading and supporting staff
- Step 3: Integrating all risk management activity
- Step 4: Promoting incident reporting
- Step 5: Involving and communicating with patients and the public
- Step 6: Learning and sharing safety lessons
- Step 7: Implementing solutions to prevent harm

For each step, there is a set of key principles and actions that organisations can take at local level to move their patient safety agenda forward. Self-assessment of an organisation's compliance with the seven steps provides a good baseline against which they can benchmark and set goals for improvement and further development. The reference guide, together with a range of tools and techniques to manage risk is available at www.npsa.nhs.uk.

Standards for Better Health

The *Standards for Better Health* (DH, 2004) are structured into seven domains made up of core and developmental standards. The standards apply to all NHS, voluntary and private organisations providing services for NHS patients. They set out the expected level of quality in terms of safety; clinical and cost-effectiveness; governance; patient focus; accessible and responsive care; care environment and amenities; and public health.

From 2005 organisations have been required to undertake a self-assessment against the core standards and make a declaration on their level of compliance, endorsed by the Trust Board — see *Table 6.1*.

Before its submission to the Healthcare Commission, the declaration is sent to the patient and public involvement forum, the local overview and scrutiny committee and the strategic health authority, who comment on the accuracy of the Trust's declaration. Compliance with the standards is a key component of the annual health check, the system for providing annual performance ratings.

The Healthcare Commission selectively inspects a sample of organisations to judge the adequacy of the evidence they have used to make their declaration. Where an organisation is unable to demonstrate that it has met the standards, an action plan is required, to show how and when they will achieve compliance.

Table 6.1. Self-assessment against core standards	
Compliant	The organisation has met the standard without any significant issues and can provide evidence of assurance
Not met	The organisation has not met the standard
Insufficient assurance	It is not clear whether the organisation is compliant as there is not enough evidence of assurance

The second report on the state of health care in England has now been published by the Healthcare Commission (2006) and highlights how organisations measure up to the *Standards for Better Health*. Further information on how organisations are performing against the standards can be accessed at www.healthcarecommission.org.uk/nationalfindings/stateofhealthcare.cfm.

Managing Risk in a Complex Organisation

This section provides a brief overview of the strategies used for delivering the patient safety agenda across one large acute care NHS organisation and gives examples of practical solutions introduced to minimise risk to patients and staff. A robust risk management system increases an organisation's capacity to handle risk efficiently leading to greater effectiveness in managing patient safety. The benefits of developing a systematic approach to the identification, assessment and management of clinical risk include a reduction in preventable patient safety incidents; better targeted staff training and education; efficient use of resources; a safer environment for patients, staff and visitors; and increased public confidence. Effective risk management requires organisations to be both proactive and reactive in sustaining improvements in patient safety.

Taking a proactive stance requires the identification and management of risk issues before actual harm occurs. For example by risk assessment of known hazards and activities, reporting near misses, learning from other organisation's failures, reviewing existing services from a safety perspective, and by sharing experiences and concerns. Clinical staff who deliver direct patient care are well placed to recognise where things can be improved and they should be actively encouraged and involved in identifying and managing risk.

Reacting in a timely and appropriate way when things go wrong is equally important in order to mitigate the degree of harm, investigate, and provide patients and staff with information as quickly as possible. This is reliant on all staff understanding their individual responsibilities for patient safety and their willingness to report incidents and respond to complaints.

Implementing the Patient Safety Agenda
Safe, quality patient care is the cornerstone of clinical governance and it is what all staff aspire to deliver. Given the wide range of national patient safety initiatives, each with their individual expectations, it is unsurprising that whilst organisations may be clear about what is expected they may be less clear about how to deliver it. The delivery of robust systems of risk management that are not too complex for staff to use, and yet ensure all national and local requirements are met is a major challenge for healthcare organisations.

What follows is a description of some of the measures developed by

Queen's Medical Centre in Nottingham (QMC) to address the challenges of reducing avoidable harm, delivering safe care, improving patient outcomes and enhancing the patient's overall healthcare experience.

Queen's Medical Centre
Queen's Medical Centre University Hospital NHS Trust is an acute teaching hospital which serves a local population of over 600,000 and between 2 and 3 million people regionally with specialist services. It has an annual income of over £300m, employs over 6500 staff and has 1100 beds, and each year it treats more than half a million inpatients and outpatients, with a further 156,000 coming through the emergency department. The Trust has four divisions: Medical; Surgical; Diagnostic and Facilities; and Women, Children and Clinical Support Services. These four divisions compromise over 40 departments and directorates.

Trust Board
Support and commitment from the Board is seen as crucial to a successful organisation wide patient safety programme. The Medical Director provides the strategic leadership and works closely with designated executive and non-executive board members to deliver all areas of governance, and to ensure an integrated approach to the management of patient safety.

Corporate Clinical Governance Team
A core team support the Medical Director at corporate level; the quality and clinical governance manager, the clinical risk lead and the clinical risk facilitator. The team is the central resource for all issues related to clinical governance. The members of the team have a clinical background which is viewed as advantageous in appreciating the complexities involved in the management of patient safety. The team enjoy strong links with non-clinical colleagues, for example the health and safety team and jointly support staff across the organisation.

The quality and clinical governance manager is tasked with managing the implementation of the organisation's strategies and policies related to clinical governance. The post holder is also responsible for establishing and leading on systems that ensure the organisation fulfils its obligation for statutory and other reporting across the range of clinical governance activities and for providing expert advice to the Trust's committees.

The clinical risk lead provides strategic leadership and is responsible for the day-to-day operational management of the patient safety programme. The post holder acts as the Trust's lead adviser on the reporting and management of all patient safety incidents and the development and delivery of an ongoing programme of training and education. Other key areas of the job include achieving compliance with national patient safety standards, supporting and facilitating safety initiatives in divisions, directorates and departments and raising the profile of risk management across and beyond the organisation.

The clinical risk facilitator has a supporting role in delivering the patient safety programme and is responsible for operationalising the team's communication strategy. The post holder is also responsible for managing the clinical incident reporting module of our risk management database, with a focus on quality improvement, implementation of local requirements and external reporting to the NPSA.

Divisions, Directorates and Departments

Each division has a forum where clinical governance activity is discussed and monitored with nominated leads responsible for ensuring safe systems and processes are in place and best practice is disseminated. Senior teams undertake peer reviews with other divisions on risk assessments and incident investigations. They act as a resource for those who seek assurances about the delivery of action plans to reduce risk, challenging where appropriate and ensuring significant risks are escalated up the organisation.

Each directorate and department has a local governance group where specialty specific risks, incidents, complaints and claims are reviewed and action is agreed and monitored. These groups will look at issues such as the quality of local induction programmes, audit results and training requirements. Each directorate and department has a nominated clinical governance co-ordinator who is a senior clinician. They play an active role on their local governance groups and are our network of patient safety champions across the organisation.

Some high-risk specialties have developed additional roles like risk facilitators for maternity services and the emergency department, and such roles are undertaken by senior clinical nurses and midwives who are given dedicated time to manage their clinical governance activity. Other key roles in the Trust with specific accountability for patient safety include all clinical directors, matrons and clinical service department managers.

Committee Structure for Clinical Governance

Figure 6.1 outlines the various committees responsible for clinical governance including risk management and how they link between local departments and the Board. There is cross representation on the committees, which improves communication and understanding and ensures the appropriate flow of information.

Risk Management Strategy

The risk management strategy is approved by the Board and sets out a clearly defined organisational structure describing the roles and responsibilities of

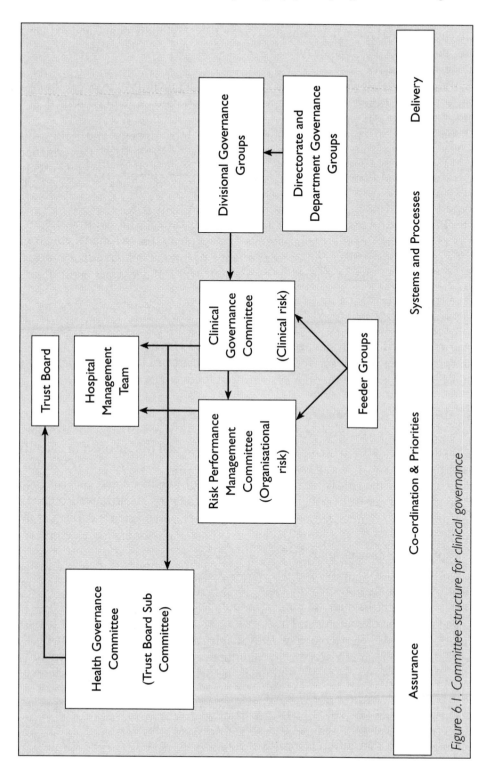

Figure 6.1. Committee structure for clinical governance

divisions, directorates, departments, committees, and individuals, and explains the process for the management of risk across the hospital. This strategy is reviewed annually.

The organisation's clinical governance development plan sets out the key governance objectives for the next 3 years (such as clinical audit priorities), and is reviewed on an annual basis.

The Clinical Governance Committee develops strategy and policy for Trust wide coordination of clinical governance. The Risk Performance Management Committee develops strategy and policy for Trust-wide management of non-clinical/organisational risk. Both these committees report to the Health Governance Committee, which is a sub committee of the Board and is responsible for providing the Board with assurance about the effectiveness of the organisation's arrangements for the management of all risk. This assurance comes from a range of internal and external sources, including accreditation reports, reviews by Royal Colleges, and audit of risk management processes.

QMC has a number of departments and professional groups responsible for different elements of the risk agenda which are geographically separated and report to different managers and directors. In recognition of the potential to fragment the overall service and create duplication of effort, we are working towards further integrating our systems for all governance activities.

Implementing Risk Management: Risk Assessment

We use a single risk assessment tool to assess all types of risk, for example, patient safety, staff safety, finances, and environmental risk. In order to quantify and prioritise our risks, a score is assigned to each risk using a 5x5 matrix. Calculation of the risk is based on assessment of likelihood and consequence. Likelihood is defined as the chances or frequency of an unwanted outcome occurring, for example, remote, likely or certain. Consequence is defined as the probable severity or impact of the unwanted outcome, for example, temporary incapacity, permanent injury or loss of a service.

The final score reflects the residual risk, after taking into account the control measures currently in place to help prevent it. Example of control measures might be staff training, new policies, assessment of competence or standardisation of equipment. The lowest score in the matrix is 2 and the highest is 25. Our risk assessment tool is available electronically and automatically calculates the total risk score. Any additional actions or controls that could be introduced to further reduce or eliminate the risks are documented together with the associated resource implications.

Because the process is partly subjective we recommend that small multi-professional groups undertake risk assessments. The diversity, skills and level of experience that different professionals can bring are an essential part of

Table 6.2. Levels at which risk can be accepted and managed		
Risk score	**Level at which risk can be managed**	**Who needs to be informed**
Less than 10	Directorate/Department	Division
10–14	Division	Risk Performance Management Committee
15–19	Risk Performance Management Committee	Hospital Management Team
20 or more	Hospital Management Team	Trust Board

testing out the subjectivity and also encourages local ownership of the risks. The residual risk escalates the process at four distinct levels as the severity increases and where there is potential for organisation-wide learning and action — see *Table 6.2.*

In order to assess and manage risk staff have access to a range of information and support to inform their risk assessments, which includes: incident and near miss data; patient feedback data; audit results; claims data; national standards (to use as a baseline); reports from external reviews and inspections; external alerts and bulletins; and access to specialist advisers.

All risks are entered onto our risk register and are performance managed at committee level. In order to appreciate and effectively manage the complete risk portfolio, clinical risks are considered alongside all other types of risk and the information used to inform the organisation's decision-making processes.

An example of a successful risk assessment submitted to our Clinical Governance Committee resulted in the recruitment of two specialist practitioners of transfusion to deliver staff education and support on all aspects of safe blood transfusion practice.

Induction, Education and Training

In order to raise staff awareness about the importance of clinical risk management, patient safety is an integral component of our corporate induction programmes. In addition to the general staff induction we also provide specific clinical induction days for all professional groups. Staff also receive a handbook of useful tips and information. Our directorate and department managers ensure specialty specific induction takes place expanding on the corporate information and providing the local context.

Ongoing training and education is delivered in a variety of formats, including the intranet, workshops on a range of topics, and presentations of case studies and lessons learned. The feedback from staff has shown us that they value the presentation of 'real event' case studies and have identified these as the most powerful way of learning and retaining the critical points. They are delivered in a non punitive way with the emphasis placed on learning

Governance in 90 minutes

Time is precious for busy clinicians, and with this in mind two identical events were held over two months entitled 'Governance in 90 Minutes'. Well-publicised in advance and introduced by the Chief Executive, the sessions attracted over 150 staff. Consultants and members of the governance team delivered short presentations of 8–10 minutes duration, covering key issues and updates. Topics included managing complaints and patient feedback, top tips for safe medication practice, blood transfusion, principles of consent and claims management. Analysis of local data was an integral part of each presentation. Copies of the presentations were made available to take away and were also posted on the intranet. The presenters were also available at the end for one-to-one discussion.

Patient safety conference:

This was a full day event with external speakers including representatives from the NPSA and the Royal College of Nursing. The Nottingham Coroner also gave an overview on the role of HM Coroner and provided much food for thought around the consequences of poor record-keeping. Facilitated workshops took place during the afternoon and included one of our ex-patients giving a first hand account of his hospital stay. Other topics included medication safety, integrated care pathways and medical devices management. The conference attracted 84 delegates from within QMC and across Nottingham and Lincolnshire, and provided an excellent forum for staff to network and share experiences; 70% of delegates completed an evaluation form and feedback was extremely positive.

Professional development programme for consultants and specialist registrars:

This two-day programme runs every 6 months and supports those clinicians responsible for the management of their services. The topics covered include:

- The Trust values
- Responding to patient feedback
- Infection control
- Managing poor performance
- Financial planning
- Managing change

Figure 6.2. Educational sessions.

and sharing experiences and how these can be translated into local practice. A selection of our educational sessions are shown in *Figure 6.2*.

Working in Partnership

The organisation has developed strong links with our regional NPSA patient safety manager who has provided on-site training in Root Cause Analysis techniques and advised on the implementation of NPSA recommendations at local level.

QMC was one of six pilot sites to implement the *Cleanyourhands* campaign aimed at getting staff and visitors to use the alcohol hand rub sited at the entraces to wards and near patients' beds, improving hand hygiene techniques and reducing the risk of infection. Following its evaluation by the NPSA, the *Cleanyourhands* campaign was rolled out across the NHS, and our infection control team supported the NPSA in this roll out with presentations of the QMC experience at both regional and national level.

The Trent Patient Safety Network is a forum for risk managers facilitated by the Strategic Health Authority which meets every quarter to discuss patient safety developments and share learning with colleagues across the region.

Trent Simulation and Clinical Skills Centre

The Trent Simulation and Clinical Skills Centre offers patient simulation based training for healthcare teams throughout the region. Using sophisticated computers to create a life like medical environment, it allows realistic scenarios to be reproduced and enacted. The adult and paediatric simulators can be set up to mimic a range of environments from operating theatres to ward settings. The focus is on inter-professional learning with emphasis on teamwork, decision-making, leadership attitudes and communication. Examples of courses provided include 'Understanding error in anaesthesia' aimed at SHO grade anaesthetic trainees and 'Life support skills and immediate management of the acutely ill ward patient' specifically targeting year 5 medical students.

The Centre Director is a consultant anaesthetist at QMC who also chairs our resuscitation committee and has close links with the clinical governance team, helping to identify specific training needs within the organisation. The Centre also has a number of clinical skills rooms designed for multidisciplinary team training, and skill-based sessions including cannulation and use of infusion devices.

Standardisation of Equipment, Systems and Processes

The instances of error should be reduced if equipment, systems and processes are standardised across an organisation or better still across the NHS. The NPSA has undertaken a considerable amount of work in this area to highlight the benefits of standardisation in terms of reducing stress, alleviating unacceptable delays in treatment and reducing patient safety incidents (NPSA, 2004). Some examples of how we have implemented both local and national initiatives include:

- A reduction in the number of different models of infusion pumps, going from 12 to 4 types, reducing the risk of unfamiliarity
- Standardisation of defibrillators reducing delays during emergency situations
- Development of a Consent to Treatment policy in line with the national model ensuring that staff moving between different hospital sites are working to the same key principles
- The standardisation of all crash-call numbers to 2222, recommended by an NPSA Safety Alert with the aim of reducing delays in accessing the emergency teams.

Open Door Policy

The quality and clinical governance team operate an 'open door' policy, where staff are free to drop in and discuss an issue, report an incident, ask for advice, or get help with a training event.

Raising Awareness

The size and complexity of the organisation presents special challenges to effective communication. We have developed and implemented a range of initiatives aimed at getting the messages about the importance of patient safety across to staff. These include:

- A patient safety page in our monthly staff newspaper outlining the latest developments
- Clinical risk posters describing key safety messages, provided in a user-friendly format
- Presentations of case studies to staff emphasising the sharing of lessons learned from incident investigations
- Bookmarks containing prompts for good record-keeping standards placed in patients' case notes
- Risk management personnel available to meet new doctors on their induction to the organisation
- Specialty specific websites on the intranet providing information about the work of various departments, for example audit results, education and training opportunities and where to access help and support
- Information leaflets distributed to all staff with their payslips showing a list of all corporate policies
- A bi-monthly bulletin sharing incidents, complaints and claims data, lessons learned and changes in practice.

Patient Involvement at QMC

The QMC Patient Partnership Group is chaired by one of our ex-patients with the goal of improving all our services to patients, carers and their families. Four sub-groups have been established and these groups operate at divisional level, and are known locally as Patient Experience Review Groups (PERGS). Each PERG consists of equal numbers of lay and staff members. They organise visits to local departments in their respective divisions to observe the delivery of direct patient care.

This initiative has facilitated the development of partnerships between patients, carers and clinical staff and supports improvements to the overall patient experience.

CNST Accreditation

Our CNST working group is chaired by the Clinical Risk Lead and has representation from clinical areas across the four divisions. The group has developed an action plan to meet the increasingly demanding national standards required by CNST. Group members champion the patient safety programme in their local areas and are committed to ensuring that we retain our compliance with the standards.

Assessment at Level 2 has a number of stages, which entails sending initial documentary evidence to the external assessors prior to their on-site visit, for example clinical audit data, information on staff induction, training records and risk assessments. The visit lasts two days and the CNST assessors meet with both the Chief Executive and the Medical Director, they interview corporate clinical governance leads, and meet clinical teams in their local areas. They also review further documentary evidence, including policies, minutes of meetings and incident data.

During our last assessment the assessors took a tour of the Trent Simulation and Clinical Skills Centre and visited our central medical equipment library. The boardroom is allocated as the assessors' base during their visit where evidence of all our patient safety initiatives is displayed.

Preparation for the CNST assessment requires a huge commitment from all areas of the organisation and is underpinned by careful preparation and effective communication. One year before the visit each directorate and department is provided with:

- A letter from the Medical Director outlining the requirements at local level
- A summary of all the standards
- Guidance on the evidence required for each standard
- A file to hold local documentary evidence
- Explanation of the process for the assessment.

The enthusiasm of all our staff for the process is evident through competition and friendly rivalry about which area will create the best evidence file! The work undertaken in individual directorates and departments is outstanding and demonstrates initiatives above and beyond the requirements of the standards, and it is a huge achievement given the backdrop of all the other competing priorities. In addition, ongoing support from the Medical Director is fundamental in keeping CNST high on the organisation's agenda and our progress is monitored by the Clinical Governance Committee with updates given to the Board at regular intervals. Our organisation has achieved compliance with the general and maternity specific standards at Level 2.

Creating a Safety Culture for Reporting

Effective incident reporting systems require simplicity, accessibility and must be easily understood by those required to use them. It is essential that staff are reassured that the system will support them if they make an error. The successful management of patient safety across the NHS requires a change in organisational culture. Such a culture must be seen to support staff when they report incidents, it must provide information on what constitutes an adverse event or clinical incident, it must provide staff with feedback from incident reporting, and ensure a positive, open and fair approach to error.

The fear of reprisals when one makes an error is a key challenge in health care, where human error has traditionally been identified as the single cause of unintentional harm. Whilst there is evidence to suggest that the tide is slowly turning and organisations are succeeding in reducing the blame culture and taking a broader 'systems' approach to patient safety incidents (NAO, 2005), anecdotal evidence from discussions with risk managers around the country acknowledge that the blame culture and associated under reporting still exists in some healthcare organisations.

Creating a culture of safety and openness takes both time and patience, and staff will only be convinced when they see first hand the way they or their colleagues are treated when mistakes are made or risk issues are raised.

Revising our Policy and Procedures Manual

At QMC we established a small multi-professional working group, comprising of both clinical and non-clinical personnel to review and revise our current arrangements for reporting incidents. As a result of the work of this group as well as the reporting requirements specified by the NPSA's National Reporting and Learning System we have considered a number of changes to our existing processes.

The revised draft policy and procedures manual was developed and tested across 16 areas of the organisation. The pilot sites provided valuable feedback which informed the final version. Comments were also sought from a variety of staff through placing a copy of the draft manual on the intranet asking for feedback electronically. The revised manual has been reproduced in an easy to follow format with key messages on the front cover reinforcing the benefits of accurate and timely reporting, and how investigations will be fair and will focus on learning and change.

Details of the revised manual were published in our newspaper, on fliers, and on designated patient safety information boards, together with dates and times of 12 planned road shows to launch the new arrangements. Specific early morning and late evening sessions were also provided so the night staff could attend. A 'go-live' date was identified when the new policy and procedures would become operational and all wards and departments received copies prior to that date in order to familiarise themselves with the contents.

Incident Reporting in Practice

Completed incident report forms are sent to the manager at local level for review and investigation, and managers are given set timescales for the follow-up to be completed. A copy of the original form is sent to a central point for collation and entry onto the organisation's risk management database. Other modules on the database include complaints, informal concerns, claims data, and the organisational risk register. Modules are linked so that, for example, when a complaint is entered, the system can flag up any incidents that have been reported for that particular patient thus prompting dialogue between relevant personnel. Integrating all our risk associated information enables closer collaboration between departments and supports improved decision-making across the organisation.

Ongoing education and awareness around incident reporting is maintained by incorporating it into our staff induction programmes, risk management training events and through a variety of written communication.

Investigation and Follow-Up

Our managers are trained on investigating incidents by the corporate risk management team as well as in partnership with the regional NPSA Patient Safety Manager. In addition there is a specific 'Manager's Section' in the Trust's Incident Reporting Manual designed to provide managers with guidance on their responsibilities following an incident. Prompts include:

- A checklist of questions to ask on receipt of an incident report form
- Examples of factors that will influence the level of investigation required
- Key issues to consider, for example has the patient been informed
- The importance of providing feedback to staff
- The need to consider if the lessons learned in one area could apply across the organisation and beyond
- Links to the NPSAs Root Cause Analysis e-learning programme.

Patient safety reports, including incident analysis and action taken to reduce risk are received and monitored by the Clinical Governance Committee on a bi-monthly cycle.

In summary, QMC supports a safety culture, which acknowledges that sometimes things go wrong, but as an organisation we learn from our mistakes and take action to put things right. We have worked hard to develop and promote robust, fair and transparent systems and processes for the reporting and management of all incidents. Training and education to explain the benefits and dispel the fears associated with incident reporting have been fundamental to our success.

Staff awareness has grown considerably over the last five years and we are now seeing a year on year increase in both the numbers and variety of reported incidents by all staff disciplines. We are not for a moment suggesting that every single incident is reported, and we acknowledge that changing staff perceptions takes a long time and we will be judged on our record. However, we do view our increased levels of reporting in a very positive light. Our analysis of trends and patterns has provided valuable data to inform our policy developments and our staff training programmes, as well as supporting proposals that require additional resources.

The next section provides a practical example of how a reported incident was investigated, managed and resulted in tangible change.

Case Study

The following case study is based on an actual clinical incident that happened in the organisation. Some aspects have been altered in order to protect the identity of the patient and staff involved. The case study describes the sequence of events leading up to the incident, the findings at investigation, the outcome and action taken — see *Box 1* below for a summary of the incident.

Box 1. Incorrect delivery of intravenous infusion

A 70-year-old male patient on a general ward was receiving intravenous fluids via a volumetric infusion pump. On completion, the senior house officer prescribed a further infusion of normal saline with added potassium chloride to be administered over 12 hours.

The registered nurse caring for the patient on the evening shift prepared the infusion, in the presence of a colleague, who provided the second check.

The infusion pump had the facility to deliver fluid at two separate rates, primary and secondary. The primary rate should have been selected to deliver the fluid over 12 hours, but the nurse incorrectly selected the secondary rate (usually used for delivering a bolus of fluid over a short period of time).

The patient received the fluid over one hour instead of 12 hours. His condition deteriorated shortly afterwards requiring intervention including diuretics, close monitoring and oxygen therapy.

Action taken following the Incident

Following the incident the following actions were undertaken:

- Help was summoned to ensure appropriate emergency measures were taken and patient safety was not further compromised
- The incident was reported promptly to the senior nursing and medical staff on duty at the time
- The patient and next of kin were informed of the error and received an apology and an explanation of the action being taken
- The incident report form was completed in accordance with Trust policy and procedures
- The specific infusion pump was withdrawn from use and sent to the Medical Equipment Service Unit for testing
- All other pumps of that particular type were withdrawn from the ward and replaced with a less complex model
- A mentor was nominated to support the nurse involved in the incident.

Investigation and Findings

An investigation was commissioned by the Medical Director and undertaken by two senior clinicians — a nurse and doctor from different specialties. The process included a review of the patient's health record, particularly the clinical entries leading up to and after the incident occurred, a review of the incident report form. The investigation team also met those staff on duty at the time of the incident and obtained written accounts of their recollections. In addition they visited the Medical Equipment Service Unit to view the infusion pump involved and ascertain whether there had been any malfunction with the device. The investigation team found that:

- Prompt and appropriate action was taken on realisation of the error
- No malfunction with the infusion pump was identified, and the manufacturer verified this following examination
- The particular model of pump had a range of operating modes and options and was more suited to critical areas than to general wards
- The nurse had not received training on the particular model of pump and was not aware of the secondary rate facility
- On the evening of the error, the nurse had selected the secondary rate by mistake, resulting in the over-infusion of fluid. This was verified by downloading the infusion pump history log
- Formal assessment of competence in the use of medical devices was not carried out systematically on that particular ward
- There were too many different types of infusions pumps in clinical areas across the Trust, making training problematic and creating the

potential for confusion and error
- The design of the infusion pump was such that the secondary rate could be selected without the requirement to verify or confirm the selection and the two buttons for the primary and secondary rates were in very close proximity to each other.

Next Steps

A written report was produced and submitted to the Trust Clinical Governance Committee. All the recommendations were endorsed and an action plan agreed. The patient and family were informed of the outcome and given an apology and explanation of how and why the incident occurred and importantly the action that was being taken by the Trust to reduce the chances of a recurrence.

The lessons learned were shared widely across the organisation and with our neighbouring Trust. The case study was anonymised and presented at the regional patient safety network (the forum for risk and governance leads) so that the key messages could be taken and applied across the patch.

Lessons Learned

The investigation identified a combination of systems failures, design failures and user error. The prompt reporting of the incident meant that a number of actions could be taken immediately, for example the withdrawal of that model of pump from the ward and the circulation of a clinical alert notice across the organisation describing how the incident could have occurred and emphasising the need for vigilance.

Timely reporting also allowed the investigation to proceed as soon as possible; whilst memories were fresh. This meant we were able to reassure the patient and his family that as an organisation, we are serious about safety and reducing risk.

This incident together with additional information from our risk management database provided the impetus to accelerate our medical devices strategy. In the two years following the incident, a significant number of changes and improvements have taken place. Some of these improvements required additional funding whilst others were cost neutral. The organisation has since been recognised as a site of good practice for the management of medical devices by our CNST assessors and the NPSA.

Key Changes Following the Incident Described in the Case Study

Education and training
- Recruitment of a medical devices trainer to coordinate education programmes across the organisation
- Weekly 'drop-in' training sessions on infusion pumps open to all clinical staff

- Purchase of database to record training and assessment of competence.

Management of infusion devices

- Expansion of our medical equipment library, improving access to the right equipment at the point of need
- Standardisation of infusion pumps across the Trust reducing the different types of pumps from 12 to 4
- Policy for the safe use of medical devices reviewed and updated.

Communication

- Monthly features on a range of medical devices in our staff newspaper
- Brightly coloured information posters in all clinical areas giving key visual reminders
- Improved intranet website, making information about all types of medical devices available to staff.

Design

- The ease with which the secondary rate could be selected on the infusion pump was of concern and resulted in installation of new software by the manufacturers. This made selection of the secondary rate a deliberate action by asking the programmer to confirm that they required this mode. This was by far the most powerful risk reducing measure, designing out the potential for harm to recur, by significantly reducing the chance of user error.

Managing Serious Untoward Incidents

When something catastrophic happens the price paid by patients can indeed be high. However, the consequences of serious untoward incidents can also have a great impact on the staff involved and the organisation. The reputation of the organisation is at stake with resultant impact on public confidence as well as the potential for significant litigation costs

A recent Department of Health publication (DH, 2000) described how serious errors had been repeated a number of times across the NHS over a period of years and in very similar circumstances because organisations were failing to learn from the past. This was tragically brought home to our hospital in 2001 with the untimely death of a young man in our care, following the maladministration of an anti-cancer drug. The circumstances of this catastrophic event resulted from a series of complex, interrelated issues and had a profound effect on the entire organisation.

A serious untoward incident (SUI) can be declared when a patient, member of the public, or a member of staff suffers serious injury, major permanent harm, unexpected death, or the risk of death or injury whilst on NHS premises, or where the actions of health service staff are likely to cause significant public concern.

Our organisation has a specific procedure to follow in the event of a SUI including immediate reporting to a Trust director. The director, in consultation with a member of the governance team will assure themselves that all immediate action has been taken, including:

- Ensuring that the area where the SUI occurred has been made safe
- If a medical device or other equipment is involved that it has been quarantined
- That the manager of the area is aware of the incident
- That an incident report form has been completed
- That the Chief Executive is informed.

As soon as practically possible, the patient (and/or) next of kin is informed that they have been involved in an SUI, what the likely consequences are and what action is being taken. In the case of patient related incidents, the first duty of the organisation is to the patient, and the requirement to establish effective channels of communication early in the process is essential. We have found that an explanation 'upfront' about what has happened and an apology goes a long way to reassuring the patient and next of kin that the organisation will be open and honest with them. From then on they must be kept informed of progress at all stages of the process.

External Reporting

Organisations are required to externally report all SUIs to the Strategic Health Authority and in the case of a patient safety incident also to the patient's general practitioner. The type of SUI may dictate that other external agencies also be notified (examples include The Health and Safety Executive, the police, the public health department).

Record Keeping

It is essential to ensure the preservation of the patient's health record following a SUI. A photocopy may need to be taken so that important information is not lost. Staff involved in the incident must be asked to document an account of their involvement whilst memories are fresh and retain it to help with writing a statement if one is required at some later stage.

All information submitted as part of the investigation of an incident is disclosable in the event of subsequent legal proceedings. As such it is crucial that staff record fact only and not opinion on the incident report form. Furthermore if they are asked to provide a statement they must be given the opportunity to ask for their professional organisation/trade union representative to give an opinion on the statement prior to it being submitted to the inquiry panel.

Media Attention
Any SUI has the potential to generate media attention and it is important to remember that patient and staff privacy and confidentiality must be preserved. All communication with the media is channelled through the head of communications for the organisation, who is skilled in managing such situations.

The Internal Inquiry
An internal inquiry panel will be established and terms of reference agreed. Membership of the panel will depend upon the nature of the SUI and may comprise of, for example, a senior consultant, (outside of the specialty where the incident occurred) the director of nursing and a member of the governance team. However, close contact with the directorate or department should be maintained throughout the inquiry. The inquiry panel also reserves the right to seek external expert advice if this is deemed appropriate.

The panel will read all the available documentation, for example the patient's health record, statements from staff, policies and procedures. They will then compile a chronology of events in order to establish the issues and circumstances surrounding the SUI. All relevant staff will be interviewed to clarify their written evidence and answer any specific questions generated from the information collected. The patient and/or relatives are also invited to meet the panel and highlight their concerns first hand. Staff are always given the opportunity to be accompanied by a friend, or a colleague acting in a personal capacity or by their professional organisation or trade union representative. All staff who are interviewed are given the opportunity to read the relevant extracts of the report that apply to them whilst it is in draft form, and are invited to comment on the accuracy of these extracts.

The final written report is submitted to the Health Governance Committee for ratification, after which it is shared with all the staff involved. The patient and/or family are given the opportunity to meet with members of the inquiry panel to hear the outcome and have their concerns answered. They receive a copy of the written report together with a formal apology from the organisation. An action plan must also be developed with the directorate/department staff and submitted to the Health Governance Committee for approval and monitoring. Staff and patients are made aware that in complex cases, the entire inquiry process make take up to six months to complete.

Support for Staff

The level of support required for the staff involved cannot be over estimated and support mechanisms need to be identified at the earliest possible time. Staff involved in a SUI receive written information explaining the stages of the inquiry and have a nominated mentor to support them through the process. It is very important that individuals continue to receive the appropriate level of help not only during, but also in the aftermath of the inquiry. It can also be therapeutic if they are involved in helping to generate solutions to mitigate future risk and in implementing the panel's recommendations.

Positive Conclusions

Whilst identifying what went wrong, why it went wrong and taking action to prevent a recurrence is the primary aim of investigating an incident, analysis often also reveals good practice within the area and this should be identified in the final written report. This will not only help to provide a balanced account of all the findings, but will help to rebuild morale in a team that will undoubtedly be feeling vulnerable (Vincent and Taylor-Adams, 2001).

Summary and Conclusions

The intention of this chapter has been to provide the reader with the national context around clinical risk management and an insight into how that translates to local implementation within a large teaching hospital. Risk management cannot be the prerogative of a small number of people in an organisation. Investment and commitment is required from the very top with active engagement of staff at all levels. These are prerequisites for a true safety culture, one which is transparent, just and accountable and where organisational learning is a routine part of everyday practice.

In comparison with healthcare in countries like the USA and indeed across other industries like aviation and nuclear power, systems for the management of clinical risk are a relatively new concept in the NHS, developing during the late 1980s (Walshe, 2001).

The full integration of all governance activities has the ability to significantly improve the way in which an organisation manages safety and reaps benefits for patients, visitors and staff.

Whilst we still have a way to go, I believe our organisation and others across the country are making considerable progress in achieving such outcomes.

This chapter relates to Queens Medical Centre University Hospital NHS Trust, which since writing has subsequently merged with Nottingham City Hospital NHS Trust to become Nottingham University Hospitals NHS Trust

References

DH (2000) *An Organisation with a Memory*. Stationery Office, London

DH (2004) *Standards for Better Health*. Stationery Office, London

Firth-Cozens J (2001) Teams, culture and managing risk. *In: Clinical Risk Management, Enhancing Patient Safety*. Vincent C, ed. BMJ Books, *London*

Healthcare Commission (2006) *State of Healthcare*. Healthcare Commission, London

NHSLA (2005) *Clinical Negligence Scheme for Trusts* https://www.nhsla.com/Claims/Schemes/CNST (accessed 10 October 2007)

NAO (2005) *A Safer Place for Patients; Learning to improve patient safety*. NAO, London

NPSA (2004) *Seven Steps to Patient Safety: The Full Reference Guide*. NPSA, London

Vincent C, Taylor-Adams S (2001) The investigation and analysis of clinical incidents. In: *Clinical Risk Management, Enhancing Patient Safety*. Vincent c, ed. BMJ Books, London

Walshe K (2001) The development of clinical risk management. In: *Clinical Risk Management, Enhancing Patient Safety*. Vincent C, ed. BMJ Books, London

CHAPTER 7

Infection Control

Annette Jeanes

Infections can cause pain, discomfort and distress. Some infections cause serious illness and suffering. A small proportion may cause death. This chapter explains the background to infection prevention and control and the principles of practice. Actions required by organisations, the public and patients are also explained although the reader should bear in mind that changes in guidance is frequent in this speciality.

A recent prevalence survey in the UK estimated that between 5.5 and 8.2% of hospitalised patients acquired an infection during their hospital stay (HIS and ICNA, 2007) *See Table 7.1*. It is known that hospitalised patients with infections have a greater risk of mortality and morbidity (Plowman et al, 1999). Patients in primary care also acquire infections but the extent of this is not clear. Some experts have estimated that 30% of healthcare associated infections (HAI) are preventable (DH and PHL, 1995). The UK has a significantly higher rate of some infections including Methicillin-resistant *Staphyloccocus aureus* (MRSA) compared to many other developed countries (Tiemersma et al, 2004).

Preventing and controlling infection is beneficial. In the past when infection was difficult to avoid it was also difficult to treat. Currently many infections are treatable with antibiotics or other treatments although many antibiotic resistant micro-organisms are emerging. A significant proportion of infections originate from the patients own microbiological flora (endogenous) and these are the most difficult to avoid. Infections which are transmitted to the patient by an external source (exogenous) are easier to avoid. There are other important factors such as the susceptibility of the individual, the dose, viability and pathogenicity of the micro-organism which affect the risk of acquiring an infection. The means of achieving a reduction of infection is based on the use of basic principles, although there are increasingly technologies and innovations which assist. The challenge in health care is to enable and ensure compliance with good infection control practice.

Background

In the UK, political reform and public investment have been responsible for much of the improvement in disease control in the past. During industrialisation

Table 7.1. Hospital-acquired infections			
Country	**Number of hospitals**	**Number of patients**	**Infection prevalence rate**
UK and Ireland (exc. Scotland)	273	75,763	7.6%
England	190	58,795	8.2%
Wales	23	5,825	6.3%
Northern Ireland	15	3,625	5.5%
Republic of Ireland	45	7,518	4.9%
HIS and ICNA (2007) The Third Prevalence Survey of Healthcare Associated Infections In Acute Hospitals 2006 — England (Summary of Preliminary Results 27th February 2007), Hospital Infection Society			

in the 19th Century, housing, sewage and water supplies were unable to cope with the influx of people to towns. Consequently, epidemics of smallpox, typhus, typhoid and cholera were common. This resulted in a series of public health reforms in the later half of the nineteenth century to control and prevent these diseases. The Public Health Service and the role of Medical Officers of Health were created. This was a predecessor of the NHS, which was established much later in 1948.

Although the role of infection control nurse was not developed until 1959, the concept and practice of using specific measures and actions to control or prevent infections is well established. The scope of infection prevention principles extends across all areas of public health and health care delivery including water supply, sewage, school health, maternal health, sexual health, food hygiene, dentists, hospitals and primary health care.

Infection prevention and control is the responsibility of everyone involved in healthcare. Whilst the healthcare workers (HCW) carry the major burden of ensuring practice is as safe as possible, visitors and patients can also contribute. The role of the infection control practitioner (ICP) is manifold and contributes to the best practice possible within the constraints of the situation. They can offer support, education, advice, leadership and other skills related to preventing and controlling infection. Normally these individuals have an infection control qualification.

Guidance and Initiatives

Public awareness of the hazards of infections has increased in recent years, particularly with the increasing prevalence of MRSA. As a consequence, the direction of public health and healthcare services in the UK has changed and there is a greater emphasis on control and prevention of infection. In 1999 the government white paper '*Saving Lives: our healthier nation*', there was a pledge to reform services which included infectious disease control. This was followed by *The NHS Plan* (DH, 2000) in which the government set out a vision of reform including 'an organisation with memory' and the introduction of national standards within health care.

In the same year a report by the National Audit Office estimated the cost of HAI in England to be over £1 billion annually (NAO, 2000). The government responded to criticism of dirty hospitals by launching a clean hospitals programme which sought to improve standards of cleaning and hygiene (DH, 2004). More than £30 million was given to NHS trusts to begin a series of sustainable improvements to hospital cleanliness and the broader patient environment. Patient Environment Action Teams (PEAT) were established and began monitoring environmental standards in hospitals.

Changes in the autonomy of the countries within the UK meant that each has separate systems and publications. Therefore for simplicity the documents primarily associated with the changes in England are used in this section. In England '*Getting ahead of the curve*' was published in 2002 (DH, 2002). This set out the strategy for infectious disease control in England. A number of other related documents followed including '*Winning ways*' (DH, 2003) which set out key areas for action including surveillance, reducing risks from devices, reducing reservoirs of infection, high standards of hygiene, prudent use of antibiotics, management and research. It also established the role of director of infection prevention and control as a strategic and operational lead responsible to the chief executive. Other guidance followed such as the Matrons charter (Jones, 2004) which clarified the role of the modern matron as pivotal in establishing a cleanliness culture. In 2005 the '*Saving lives*' delivery programme was launched and provided a delivery programme which included 'high impact interventions' e.g. a central venous care programme. Whilst the emphasis was initially on hospital care, subsequently community focused guidance was produced (DH, 2006) which gave a framework for improvement to non-acute and community providers. In the same year '*Going further faster*' (DH, 2006) gave further guidance on improvement programmes. Finally, the Health Act of 2006 established a legal obligation for healthcare providers to reduce and prevent infection and in the code of practice gave detailed guidance for infection prevention and control practice implementation.

It has been argued that an emphasis on meeting performance targets in the UK coupled with increased patient throughput and bed occupancy has increased the risk of infection to patients (Cunningham et al, 2006). This is twinned with finite resources and an increasing public expectation. Consequently there is the potential for a shortfall in healthcare workers performance and public satisfaction. This in turn has led to litigation and compensation claims.

Actions to reduce the risk of infection are increasingly based on evidence rather than ritual. In 2001, Pratt et al published the result of a government sponsored study to develop evidence based infection control guidelines. This comprehensive publication critically reviewed the evidence base for infection control practices and made recommendations for practice. This has subsequently been reviewed and updated (Pratt et al, 2007).

In the US when patients groups became dissatisfied by the efforts of health care providers to reduce the risks of infection, their actions resulted in change. The campaign '*Saving a hundred thousand lives*' was led by the Institute for Healthcare Improvement. The result of the campaign showed that by utilizing evidence based interventions, infections could be reduced. 'Bundles' of evidence based interventions were used to prevent and reduce infections (Berriel-Cass et al, 2006). Some healthcare interventions such as inserting a urinary catheter or a central venous catheter are known to carry a significant risk of infection. Simple strategies such as training inserters, using a sterile insertion technique and removing the device as soon as possible, were effective in reducing infections.

Successful strategies have been used elsewhere particularly in northern Europe. In the Netherlands the 'seek and destroy' approach was used to reduce and control rates of MRSA. Patients were screened for the presence of MRSA on their skin or in their nose on admission to hospital. If the result was positive, patients were isolated and treated with antiseptic washes and nasal antibiotic. Staff also received treatment if they were screened positive. This contributed to a low rate of MRSA prevalence in the Netherlands and the control of MRSA transmission (Vos et al, 2005). Although this approach has been criticised (Gebhardt, 2003), similar approaches have been used successfully in the UK (Schelenz et al, 2005).

In Geneva, work by Pittet et al found that infections decreased by improving hand hygiene compliance with the introduction of alcohol based decontaminants and monitoring compliance and feed-back (Pittet et al, 2000). Similar work in the UK (McGuckin et al, 2001; Rao, 2002) preceded the '*Cleanyourhands*' campaign in England, which was aimed at improving hand hygiene in healthcare (Storr, 2005).

Further work produced compelling evidence in the 1980s that surveillance of infections in hospital twinned with control activities led to reductions in infection rates (Haley el al, 1985). Successful components of the programme included adequate staffing of infection control practitioners (one full-time infection control nurse for 250 beds), and reports to the surgeons of their infection rates. Targeted surveillance particularly of surgical operations was cost effective and led to the development of the National Infection Surveillance (NIS) system in the US. A similar system the National Scheme for Surveillance of Surgical Site Infection has been set up in England with similar effects (McDougall et al, 2004).

World Health Organisation

The World Health Organisation (WHO) has recognised the impact of healthcare associated infections. In '*Clean care is better care*' (Pittet el al, 2006) WHO launched a global patient safety challenge which commenced with interventions to reduce healthcare associated infection. These included the provision of water, sanitation, waste management, blood safety, injection safety and the promotion of hand hygiene.

Industry

Industry and other innovators have also joined this quest for improvements. Technologies such as silver and antibiotic impregnated devices, micro fibres and steam for cleaning, special antibacterial coating for work surfaces and equipment are a few examples. Unfortunately no one item or intervention will prevent all HAI. Prevention and control is more complex and is largely dependent on the actions and behaviour of healthcare workers, patients and to some extent visitors. Generally the appropriate responses are grouped as principles of infection prevention and control which ensures a consistent approach.

Principles of Infection Prevention and Control

The principles of infection prevention and control are relatively straightforward. The interpretation may vary from one organisation to another and many organisations have comprehensive policy or guideline documents. The basic principles of infection prevention and control are:

- Standard precautions
- Hand hygiene
- Personal hygiene
- Personal protective equipment (PPE)
- Isolation, separation or cohorting
- Sharps and waste management,
- Asepsis
- Reprocessing of instruments and equipment
- Clean environment and equipment
- Surveillance and monitoring

Standard Precautions

Standard precautions (formerly known as universal precautions) are a precautionary approach to all care and treatment of patients regardless of the perceived risk of infection (CDC, 1987; Lynch, 1987; Lynch et al, 1990). This applies to both staff and patients. It includes the use of PPE, aseptic technique, hand hygiene, environmental controls, reprocessing of equipment and safe handling of blood and body substances. Additional precautions are required when there is a particular risk of transmission of infection which may not be encompassed by standard precautions for example airborne infections.

Hand Hygiene

Hand hygiene includes hand washing with soap and water and hand decontamination with alcohol or other types of hand decontaminant. Hands are an important vector in the transmission of infection in health care (Larson, 1988). Cleaning hands, particularly before and after patient contact reduces the risk of transmission of infection (Pittet el al, 2000). To ensure effective hand hygiene health care workers should keep nails short and free of nail polish, avoid watches or jewellery and roll up sleeves whilst they work (RCN, 2005). Hands should be washed or decontaminated before and after each patient contact, when hands have become soiled and before clean or sterile areas are touched (Boyce and Pittet, 2002). The method used is important. The Ayliffe six stage method of hand washing is recommended as it covers all areas of the hands (Ayliffe et al, 2000). This is particularly useful in areas such as theatres. Alcohol decontaminants evaporate fast and other techniques may be used to cover important areas of the hands, i.e. finger tips first (Jeanes, 2005).

Personal Hygiene

Personal hygiene is also important as micro-organisms may be present on the skin or clothing of healthcare workers, patients and relatives. Reducing the number of micro-organisms present by washing and maintaining clean clothing is believed to contribute to infection reduction. General cleanliness is also desirable in reducing the number of transmissible micro organisms on the body including nails, hair and skin (Parker, 2004).

Personal Protective Equipment (PPE)

Personal Protective equipment (PPE) is used to protect the patient and/or the healthcare worker from infection transmission. This includes disposable gloves, aprons, gowns, masks, visors or goggles.

Gloves — the purpose of gloves is to prevent hands becoming contaminated and to prevent the micro-organisms on the hands of the health care worker contaminating the patient. The type of glove selected should be determined by the task and the relative risks (ICNA, 2002). Sensitivity to latex occurs in staff and patients, so non latex alternatives should be available and gloves should be removed as soon as possible (MDA, 1996). Hand hygiene is still required when gloves are worn.

Aprons and gowns — aprons and gowns are worn to protect the health care worker becoming contaminated during patient contact and to protect the patient from the contaminants on the health care workers clothing or body. In some instances suits or overalls may also be appropriate. Many of these items are disposable and should not be reused. Others are reusable, e.g. theatre gowns, and these may be laundered to remove and destroy contaminants and micro organisms.

Isolation — separation or cohorting are used to protect patients who are particularly vulnerable to infection or to limit the contacts of patients with transmissible infections or diseases. Isolation is ideally a single room with an en-suite toilet and shower. Purpose built isolation facilities may have specialist air handling systems which filter air flows. These are usually positive pressure or negative pressure facilities. In positive pressure isolation rooms, air is pushed out of the room into the adjoining corridor. This prevents potentially contaminated air reaching the patient and is used for patients vulnerable to infection. In negative pressure isolation rooms' air is sucked into the room and discharged away from the facility. This ensures any infectious organisms in the air do not reach surrounding patients and staff. Separation may involve having separate waiting areas for potentially infected and non-infectious clients or sometimes specific wards and care facilities for those with the same infection. Cohorting normally refers to grouping of people with the same infection.

In some circumstances isolation though desirable is not possible due to limited isolation facilities or because there are insufficient staff to care for the patient safely. In these instances staff should risk assess and prioritise whilst utilising resources available. Managers should be alerted to the risks to patients and staff when isolation is not possible. The discussion leading to the decisions and actions should be documented.

The type of isolation is dependent on the mode of transmission of the micro-organism. Each disease has transmission characteristics and some may be transmitted in more than one way. The common modes of transmission are contact, droplet, airborne, feaco-oral, and vector. Vertical transmission of an infection from infected mother to newborn infant can also occur.

Common Modes of Transmission:

Contact — this includes direct contact and indirect contact. Direct contact involves close physical contact and includes touching, kissing, sexual contact and contact with secretions. In healthcare hand hygiene and glove usage are normally the primary methods of preventing direct contact transmission.

Indirect contact usually involves items in the environment which have become contaminated and come into contact with a susceptible individual. These are known as fromites and include handles, rails, tables, beds, toys and medical instruments. Optimal cleanliness and maintenance of surfaces and equipment can reduce this form of transmission (Rampling et al, 2001).

Droplet — droplets of liquid containing micro-organisms can be generated when people with an infection, cough, sneeze and talk. Some medical procedures such as bronchoscopy also produce droplets. Droplets are relatively heavy and do not remain airborne for long, rapidly falling to the ground but close contact may allow contamination of the eye nose and mouth of those attending. Face masks and goggles are normally used as protective barriers.

Airborne — high velocity coughing and sneezing expels aerosolised liquid from the respiratory tract and large numbers of bacteria or viruses into the air. The liquid rapidly evaporates leaving any organism originally present. This is called a droplet nucleus. Droplet nuclei settle so slowly that they remain airborne in occupied spaces and circulate on air currents. Ventilation or air exchanges dilute and eventually remove them. High filtration masks and respirators are required for close patient contact in patients with highly infectious pathogenic diseases.

Feaco-oral transmission — this occurs when contaminated food or fluid enters the digestive tract. This may follow poor hygiene during food preparation, inadequate water supply treatment and in some instances food such as shell fish which is contaminated. Measures such as thorough cooking, storage at adequate temperatures and optimal hygiene precautions during food handling are some to the measures which can be used.

Vector borne transmission is associated with animals or insects which by biting or shedding the micro-organisms spread the disease. Vectors include mosquitoes, flies, ticks, dogs and include diseases such as malaria, West Nile virus and dengue fever.

Safe Handling of Sharps

Any sharp instrument may cause injury but commonly devices such as hypodermic needles, scalpels and glass ampoules are referred to as 'sharps'. These devices may become contaminated during use, commonly with blood. This poises a potential risk of transmission of blood borne infections such as hepatitis B and C and HIV. Some procedures carry a particular risk to health care workers such as venesection and cannulation as these are hollow bore needles and may contain blood. Poor disposal of equipment following use is a hazard which may also affect patients who may be injured.

Disposal of Waste

In the UK waste management and handling is governed by stringent regulations, which includes segregation of waste into waste streams and disposal. Some types of waste are particularly hazardous including sharps, radioactive, pharmaceutical and infectious waste. These require specific processes and facilities to render them safe.

Asepsis

Asepsis in the clinical setting aims to minimise the presence of pathogenic micro-organisms. Aseptic technique is used to protect the patient from the introduction of infection and can be used in a variety of settings. Some situations and procedures increase the potential for the introduction of micro-organisms to the patient such as surgery, insertion of devices and management of extensive burns. Aspetic technique includes:

- Ensuring the area where the procedure is to take place is as clean as possible
- Ensuring as little disruption occurs during the procedure which would lead to air turbulence and dust distribution
- Cleaning hands before and at times during the procedure if contamination occurs
- Using sterile equipment
- Minimising contamination of the site by use of sterile gloves or forceps or by not touching sterile parts of the equipment (non-touch technique).

The highest levels of asepsis are used in operating theatres. A series of measures including frequent air exchange, air filtration, sterile drapes, sterile equipment, sterile surfaces, surgical scrubbing, use of disinfectants and separation of sterile and non sterile fields are taken. Staff wear clean low lint theatre garb, hair is covered and further PPE is applied by operators. This all contributes to a reduction in micro organisms near the patient. In other clinical areas or situations, similar levels of asepsis may not be achievable. In these, hand hygiene, use of sterile equipment twinned with the use of sterile gloves and or a non touch technique are used for other procedures such as urinary catheterisation and wound care.

Reprocessing of Instruments and Equipment
Instruments and equipment may be vectors of micro organisms and inadequate decontamination has been linked with outbreaks of infection such as tuberculosis (Ramsey et al, 2002). It is essential to decontaminate reusable equipment between patients. The processes include cleaning, disinfection and sterilisation. Cleaning with detergent and water removes much visible contamination but does not destroy micro organisms. Disinfection uses chemicals or heat to substantially reduce the number of organisms on the equipment. Sterilisation is usually done by steam at high temperatures. The standard of reprocessing is governed by a number of comprehensive documents which are intermittently updated (NHS, 2003). These aim to maintain consistency and efficacy of processes. Some equipment is single use and should not be reused or reprocessed.

Clean Environment and Patient Equipment
Healthcare facilities should be clean in order to reduce the risk of transmission of infection. There is a potential for transmission of micro organisms when a contaminated surface or object comes into contact with the people in the environment. There is little evidence that surfaces such as floors and walls are a particular source of

infection. However clean floors and walls are aesthetically pleasing. A visibly clean environment gives the impression of an organisation which delivers a good quality of care. Cleaning standards and methods in UK health establishments are specified in guidance and are subject to regular monitoring (DH, 2002; NHS Estates, 2004). One of the difficulties encountered in achieving the required standards is the condition and design of facilities which may be difficult to clean and may appear shabby.

Surveillance and Monitoring
Surveillance of HAI is useful in understanding the incidence of infections in order that improvement to practice can be undertaken. The incidence of HAI is used as an indicator of performance. Some surveillance of surgical site infection is mandatory. National surveillance enables benchmarking and informs patient choice. In England the Surgical Site Infections Service was established in 1997, similar systems operate in Scotland, Northern Ireland and Wales

Other surveillance of MRSA bacteraemia and *Clostridium difficile* also gives comparable data. Much surveillance which takes place in healthcare establishments is based on laboratory findings. Some establishments have comprehensive surveillance systems and are able to feedback regular information to the organisation and individual areas. This is particularly helpful in engaging clinicians and ensuring ownership and has proven to be successful in reducing infection rates (Wilson et al, 2006). However, if the data is not ready available then it may involve considerable effort by people to collect it.

Active screening of patients for MRSA and other micro-organisms may also be undertaken to determine prevalence and transmission. This can be useful as a control method as a patient with the micro-organism can be isolated and treated.

The Role of Healthcare Professional and Organisations
Preventing harm by reducing or preventing infection requires the participation of all healthcare staff. The Health Act 2006 requires healthcare providers to adhere to best practice and organisations have to account for any failures. The Healthcare Commission (HCC) is the regulator associated with these standards.

Much infection control is not complex, for example maintaining good hand hygiene. However ensuring compliance and maintaining principles of infection control can be difficult. The culture of the organisation affects the behaviour of the staff. If good infection control practice is not valued it is unlikely that staff will maintain good practice. Therefore a culture of optimal infection prevention is important (DHSSPI, 2006).

Organisation of Infection Control

The chief executives of healthcare organisations are ultimately responsible for infection control standards. The role of ensuring infection control practice is optimal is delegated to the Director of Infection Prevention and Control (DIPC), who is responsible for the infection control team in the organisation. The composition of infection control teams varies according to the size and requirements of the organisation.

Within organisations leadership and commitment to improvement is important in delivering the infection control and prevention strategy. Unfortunately there have been a number of failures related to organisational failure for example the Stoke Mandeville outbreak of *Clostridium difficile* (Healthcare Commission, 2006). The reviews and lessons learnt from numerous events have led to the development of a large body of work which guides organisations in how they should respond. This is normally produced with the professional organisations of infection control experts such as the Hospital Infection Society and the Infection Control Nurses Association. These are often guidance and lack the compulsion or resources which organisations would find useful for implementation.

In the current NHS, trusts increasingly compete to attract patients. Public confidence in healthcare delivery is affected by adverse reports. Therefore trusts aspire to meet performance targets, avoid poor press coverage, complaints and litigation. This will be assisted by a culture of openness and ownership by the trust board. To obtain a clear picture of performance some form of monitoring is required which will enable an evaluation of progress.

In each healthcare organisation clear structures and processes allow delivery of strategies and plans. This should include elements of clinical governance and risk. It should also include an equitable and pragmatic response to non compliance or failure.

Buildings and Facilities

Infection control and prevention should begin at the design stage of any facility designed for healthcare delivery. The Department of Health produces health building notes (HTN) which identify best practice in planning and design and Health building memoranda (HTM) which specify standards for components for healthcare providers, planners and builders (DH, 2005). During any building the disruption is a risk to nearby patients and precautions are required to minimise the risk of *Aspergillus* in particular (Noskin and Peterson, 2001).

Maintenance of building and facilities contributes to infection control and prevention. Facilities must be easy to clean and keep clean, must minimise the risk of infection transmission such as legionnaires in showerheads or pipe work (DH, 2006). Heating and ventilation systems require regular planned maintenance particularly in clean rooms and theatres. Areas such as therapy pools, laboratories, endoscopy units, mortuaries, sterile services departments all have separate maintenance guidelines. Performance in achieving standards should be monitored regularly and any failures or potential risk should be identified to managers.

Equipment also requires maintenance and part of that will be effective cleaning and decontamination. Purchasing equipment which is easy to clean and maintain is crucial and should be part of the specification requirement. Equipment which is returned to manufacturers or companies and that which requires maintenance should always be carefully decontaminated before it is handled by engineers or technicians to prevent transmission of micro organisms (DH, 2003).

Services

Many services may be offered by healthcare providers, but the key ones are:

- Catering
- Cleaning
- Laundry or linen.

Catering

Food hygiene is a risk wherever it is undertaken and healthcare is no different. Food hygiene standards and regulations apply to healthcare organisations in the same way as restaurants or manufacturers elsewhere (Statutory Instrument 2006). Some patients such as the immunocompromised are particularly susceptible to contamination of food and may require particular care.

Cleaning

Cleaning standards in the NHS are standardised in the cleaning manual and national standards. In health care some areas require a higher level of cleanliness and cleaning frequency than others. An example is operating theatres compared to administrative staff offices. Monitoring of standards should be undertaken regularly to ensure the highest standards are achieved. Cleaning schedules should reflect the requirements of areas and the methods used should reflect best practice. Perception of cleanliness is important and an effort should be made to ensure spillage and marks are rapidly removed, bins emptied and toilets cleaned when they become unsightly between cleans. Staff have to take ownership of areas and liaise with cleaning staff to identify requirements and any changing needs. Where equipment is present it is helpful to clarify whose role it is to clean it and the method and frequencies required.

Laundry

Infected and contaminated laundry is a potential source of micro-organisms. Specific standards are available in national guidance which details the handling, securing and disinfection of linen (DH, 1995).

Practice and Policies

Most healthcare organisations will have infection control manuals or national guidelines. These act as a resource and reference point but require regular updating as guidance changes frequently. Policies associated with specific micro-organisms such as MRSA and *Clostridium difficile* may be adapted from the latest available guidelines. Antibiotic policies may require considerable negotiation before agreement is reached.

It is important that clear systems and processes are available and understood, particularly in relation to outbreaks of infection and lapses in compliance with guidance. Policies alone will not change behaviours and therefore education and training is required for all healthcare staff in basic principles of infection prevention and control. Role models and champions are also useful.

Quality assurance is required which includes audits, monitoring and reviews of infection control practice and responses to challenges. Infection control committees serve as a focus for this work and also provide an opportunity for engagement of key clinical and managerial staff in achieving the infection control agenda. A strategy of implementation of an annual plan is helpful in delivering change.

Staff

All healthcare workers require occupational health screening to ensure they are not at risk of infection and also that they do not carry transmissible infections. Particularly blood borne virus and tuberculosis. Staff who are ill should not come to work particularly if they have an infection.

Infection control principles should be taught to staff on commencing employment and regularly updated. Infection control advice should be available for any queries or to deal with any incidents.

Managers should provide staff with uniforms if necessary and adequate facilities to change and shower. If possible laundering of uniforms should be undertaken by the employer rather than staff taking dirty uniforms home (RCN, 2005).

The Role of the Public and Patients

The public and patients have an important role in infection prevention and control. Unfortunately it is often not until the public enter into the healthcare system that they recognise the need. It is also difficult to ensure there is a balanced response in a busy healthcare environment when resources are limited and throughput sometimes rapid. The perception of risk particularly to untidiness or lack of cleanliness may be out of proportion to the real danger. However the objective eye of a patient or visitor may be invaluable in identifying practice which goes unnoticed or unchallenged by staff (Jeanes, 2005). Challenging poor practice is difficult particularly when a patient is in a dependent role. So mechanisms should allow feedback to healthcare providers such as PALS, comments cards, and other forms of feedback ensure an easier process.

Information

The information for patients and public may vary according to the organisation. Web based information systems are common. In the UK, the Health Protection Agency and NHS Direct have particularly helpful sites. Many organisations now publish information on infection rates and other performance information. The mandatory reporting of MRSA and *Clostridium difficle* are available on the internet and give comparison data for other organisations. Under the Freedom of Information Act the public may request details of results and performance and increasingly clinicians are aware of the facts and figures and are prepared to discuss them in detail.

Preparation

If possible the public should be aware of the issues of their local healthcare providers and any successes or failures encountered. If there is a choice of facilities and treatments beyond the local area then infection control performance may be a factor. Rates of infection and mortality are difficult to interpret. Some facilities may be a single well funded speciality with low risks whilst others may be dealing with a complex case mix, limited resources multiple risk factors. If there is time and opportunity open days, patient's forums or visiting, offer an opportunity for a preview. Listening to the stories and experiences of patients is also helpful although it should be remembered that stories where everything went well tend to be quite boring and receive less attention.

Action

The Patients Association have produced a number of documents and led a number of campaigns relating to the prevention of infection. The Patients Association '*Ten Top Tips*' (Patients Association, 2006) offers practical and simple advice particularly about how to help prevent infections in hospital. It also encourages a proactive rather than passive stance by patients in asking questions, improving their hygiene and organising visitors. Simple signs to check on the infection control in a healthcare environment are:

- Are staff washing or decontaminating their hand regularly?
- Do staff change disposable gloves between patients?
- Are surfaces and equipment which come into regular contact with patients visibly clean?
- Is equipment cleaned between patients e.g. couch, blood pressure cuff, commode.

Patients can improve their hygiene and reduce their risk of infection by:

- Washing or decontaminating hands frequently and particularly after using the toilet and before eating.
- Bathing, showering or washing at least daily and particularly just before surgery
- Avoiding interference with dressings and devices

The public can contribute to infection prevention and control in healthcare establishments by:

- Not visiting in hospitals when suffering from an infection
- Washing or decontaminating hands before and after visiting
- Minimising any disruption to cleaning staff and ensuring cleaning can take place.

References

Ayliffe GAJ, Fraise AP, Geddes AM, Mitchell K (2000) *Control of Hospital Infection: A practical handbook. 4th edn.* Arnold, London

Berriel-Cass D, Adkins FW, Jones P, Fakih MG (2006) Eliminating nosocomial infections at Ascension Health. *Jt Comm J Qual Patient Saf* **32**(11): 612-20

Boyce JM, Pittet D (2002) Guideline for handhygiene in healthcare settings: recommendations of the healthcare infection control practices advisory committee and the HICPAC/SHEA/APIC/IDSA hand hygiene task force. *Infect Control Hosp Epidemiol* **23**(12): S3-40

Centre for Disease Control (1987) Recommendations for prevention of HIV transmission in health-care settings. *MMWR* **36**(2S): 1S-18S

Cunningham JB, Kernohan WG, Rush T (2006) Bed occupancy, turnover interval and MRSA rates in Northern Ireland. *Br J Nurs* **15**(6): 324-328

DH and Public Health Laboratory service (1995) *Hospital Infection Control. Guidance on the control of infection in hospitals.* The Hospital Infection Working Group of the Department of Health and Public Health Laboratory Service. Stationary Office, London

DH (1995) *Hospital Laundry Arrangements for Used and Infected Linen.* DH, London

DH (2000) *The NHS Plan: a plan for investment, a plan for reform.* DH, London

DH (2002) *Getting ahead of the curve: a strategy for combating infectious diseases (including other aspects of health protection).* DH, London

DH (2002) *NHS standard service level specification cleaning.* DH, London

DH (2003) *Winning Ways: Working together to seduce healthcare associated Infection In England report from the chief medical officer.* DH, London

DH (2003) *Management of medical devices prior to repair, service or investigation.* DH, London

DH (2004) *Towards cleaner hospitals and lower rates of infection: A summary of action*. DH, London

DH and NHS Estates (2005) *Health building notes and health technical memoranda*. DH, London

DH (2005) *Saving Lives: a delivery programme to reduce healthcare associated infections including MRSA*. DH, London

DH (2006) *Essential steps to safe, clean care: reducing healthcare associated infections. The delivery programme to reduce healthcare associated infections (HCAI) including MRSA*. DH, London

DH Estates (2006) *The control of legionella, hygiene 'safe' hot water, cold water and drinking systems. Part A: Design Installation and testing*. DH, London

DH (2006) *Going further faster: Implementing the saving Lives delivery programme*. DH, London

DH (2006) *Changing the culture: An Action plan for the prevention and control of healthcare associated infections in Northern Ireland (2006/2009)*. DHSSPI, Belfast

DH (2006) *The Health Act 2006: Code of practice for the prevention and control of healthcare associated infections*. DH, London

Gebhardt DOE (2003) MRSA in the Netherlands: preventive measure raises a moral issue. *J Med Ethics* **29**: 212

Haley RW, Culver DH, White JW et al (1985) The efficacy of infection surveillance and control programs in preventing nosocomial infections in US hospitals. *Am J Epidemiol* **121**(2): 182-205

Healthcare Commission (2006) I*nvestigation into outbreaks of Clostridium difficile at Stoke Mandeville hospital, Buckinghamshire hospitals NHS Trust*. Healthcare Commission, London

HIS and ICNA (2007) *The Third Prevalence Survey of Healthcare Associated Infections In Acute Hospitals 2006 - England [Summary of Preliminary Results 27th February 2007]*. Hospital Infection Society, London

ICNA (2002) *Protective clothing principles and guidance*. ICNA, London

Jeanes A (2005) Using alcohol hand rubs. *Nursing Times* **101**(28): 28-9

Jeanes A (2005) Keeping hospitals clean: how nurses can reduce health-care associated infection. *Prof Nurse* 20(6): 35-7

Jones E (2004) *A matrons charter: An Action plan for cleaner hospitals*. DH, London

Larson E (2003) A casual link between handwashing and risk of infection? Examination of the evidence. *Infect Control Hosp Epidemiol* **9**: 28-36

Lynch P, Jackson MM,Cummings MJ, Stamm WE (1987) Rethinking the role of isolation pratices in the prevention of nosocomial infections. *Ann Intern Med* **107**: 243-246

Lynch P, Cummings MJ, Roberts PL et al (1990) Implementing and evaluating a system of generic infection precautions: body substance isolation. *Am J Infect Control* **18**: 1-2

MDA (1996) *Latex sensitisation in the healthcare setting (use of latex gloves)*. MDA, London

McDougall C, Wilson J, and Leong G (2004) The National Scheme for Surveillance of Surgical Site Infection in England. *JOODP* **1**(9): 12-17

McGuckin M, Waterman R, Storr IJ et al (2003) Evaluation of a patient-empowering hand hygiene programme in the UK. *JHI* **48**(3): 222-7

NAO (2000) *The Management and Control of Hospital Acquired Infection in Acute NHS Trusts in England*. The Stationary office, London

NHS Estates (2003) *A guide to the decontamination of re-useable surgical instruments*. DH, London

NHS Estates (2004) *The NHS Healthcare cleaning manual*. DH, London

Noskin GA, Peterson LR (2001) Engineering Infection Control through facility design. *Emerg Infect Dis* 7(2): 354-7

Parker L (2004) Infection control: maintaining the personal hygiene of patients and staff. *Br J Nurs* **13**(8): 474-8

Patients Association (2006) *Ten top tips to using your patient power in Infection Control – Is it only skin deep?* Patients Association, London

Pittet D, Hugonnet S, Harbarth S et al (2000) Effectiveness of a hospital-wide programme to improve compliance with hand hygiene. Infection Control Programme. *Lancet* **356**(9238):1307-12

Pittet D, Allegranzi B, Storr J et al (2006) Clean care is safer care: the global Patient Safety Challenge. *Int J Infect Dis* **10**(6): 419-24

Plowman R, Graves N, Griffin M et al (1999) *The Socio-economic Burden of Hospital Acquired Infection, Vols I, II, III and executive summary*. PHLS, London

Pratt RJ, Pellowe C, Loveday HP et al (2001) The epic Project: Developing National Evidence-based Guidelines for Preventing Healthcare associated Infections. Phase 1: Guidelines for Preventing Hospital-acquired Infections. *J Hosp Infection* **47**(Supplement): S1-S-82

Pratt RJ, Pellowe CM, Wilson JA et al (2007) National Evidence-Based Guidelines for Preventing Healthcare-Associated Infections in NHS Hospitals in England. *J Hosp Infection* **65S**: S1-S64.

Rampling A, Wiseman S, Davis L et al (2001) Evidence that hospital hygiene is important in the control of methicillin-resistant *Staphylococcus aureus*. *J Hosp Infect* **49**(2): 109-16

Ramsey AH, Oemig TV, Massey JP, Torok TJ (2002) An outbreak of brochoscopy-related mycobacterium tuberculosis infection due to lack of bronchoscope leak testing. *Chest* **121**(3): 976-81

Rao G, Jeanes A, Osman M et al (2005) Marketing hand hygiene in hospitals — a case study. *J Hosp Infect* **50**(1): 42-7

RCN (2005) *Good practice in infection prevention and control: guidance for nursing staff. Wipe it out RCN campaign on MRSA*. RCN, London

Storr J (2005) The effectiveness of the national cleanyourhands campaign. *Nursing Times* **101**(8): 50-1

Schelenzs S, Tucker D, Georgen C et al (2005) Significant reduction of endemic MRSA acquisition and infection in cardiothoracic patients by means of an enhanced targeted infection control programme. *J Hosp Infect* **60**(2): 104-10

Tiemersma EW, Bronzwaer SL, Lyytikainen O et al (2004) European Antimicrobial Resistance Surveillance System Participants. *Emerg Infect Dis* **10**(9): 1627-34

Vos M C, Ott A, Verbrugh HA (2005) Successful Search and Destroy Policy for Methicillin resistant Staphylococcus aureus in the Netherlands. *J Clin Microbiol* **20**(3):34-35

Wilson APW (2006) Reduction in wound infection by wound surveillance with post discharge follow-up and feed back. *Br J Surg* **93**(5): 630-638

CHAPTER 8

Finding Patient Safety Information in a Digital World

Ross Scrivener

This chapter looks at the growing number of patient safety resources available online. This rapid growth risks increasing information overload and reducing our ability to find what we need. We introduce mind mapping as a prerequisite to making the best use of the most credible resources available. One form of mapping plots resources by location and type of support to be found there. Another map captures the relationships between patient safety concepts and issues. Both maps can help intrepid explorers cover the developing information landscape more thoroughly.

Mapping Patient Safety

We live in an increasingly digitised society. The Internet offers the prospect of information available 24/7. With an Internet connection and without recourse to physical libraries, we can access government policy documents, primary research and other forms of synthesised clinical evidence.

We can also access the expertise of people through discussion lists and other communities of practice or view the opinions of individuals as they publish their own weblogs (Wikipedia, 2005a).

The Internet has added a new dimension, to what some call 'extelligence' (Cohen and Stewart, 1997), the cumulative 'cultural capital' that surrounds us in the form of books, DVDs, broadcasts, folk tales and the like. However, it has also underlined a deep paradox at the heart of our Information Age. We need to be familiar with the information landscape before we can utilise it, and if we explore it before we are familiar with it we are going to get hopelessly lost.

If we are going to resolve the paradox we need to acquire a range of skills usually grouped under the label 'information literacy'. This term covers the ability to diagnose an information need and structure an intelligent question. When confronted with a problem or a decision we need to gather intelligence of some sort to help us solve the problem or weigh up options. Faced with the size, mutability and maze of the Internet we need a particular type of guide. We need a map.

Mapping techniques can help us to get our bearings in the bewildering information landscape opening up before us (Scrivener, 2002; Dale, 2003). By focusing on an area of interest, like patient safety, we can screen out much of the noise and distractions inherent in web-based searches while developing our understanding of this foreign terrain.

Mind mapping is one particular mapping technique (see *Figure 8.1*). A mind map consists of a central word or concept, from which branches are drawn radiating outward to other ideas relating to that word (Buzan and Buzan, 2006). These branches are labelled, and these 'child words' can branch again into sub-topics. Colour and images can be used to show connections and highlight relationships.

Our first mind map of patient safety is neither exhaustive nor encyclopaedic. We have used certain criteria in what we show on our mind map. We do not cover journals or sites that require paid subscriptions. We hope that we have covered sites, which, due to their provenance, or their critical acceptance within the health service community, provide the foundation for information research. It is intended as an adaptive tool designed to help us deepen our knowledge of where things are and our understanding of the uses to which these resources can be put.

Our mind map has several main branches: research, policy, patient safety tools, learning and networks. The research arm has two subsidiary arms: reviews of the evidence base such as that provided by systematic reviews and centres engaged in primary research — studies that present the results of original research. The branch labelled 'gateways' highlights places where you can find more quality-controlled information. The first mind map plots locations but this is not the only use of mind maps. While this chapter will use the first map to navigate around significant online resources it does not give the user any sense of the kinds of patient safety issues and concerns they are likely to find on the journey.

The second mind map (see *Figure 8.2*) covers some of the current themes of patient safety research and policy. We have given prominence to the debate around what constitutes a safety culture. This debate is being fuelled by complimentary fields such as human factors engineering and lessons learned from other high-risk industries outside of healthcare such as aviation. Many tools have been developed as a result of this cross-fertilization and some of these will feature in this text. The map shows the growing range of patient safety tools and strategies to reduce harm. On one side are the numerous uses of information and communication technology and on the other the active participation of patients and the public in averting harm. But so much remains to be discovered. For example, most of what is known about patient safety incidents is from studies of acute care settings. Little is known about the nature or extent of harm in other settings such as primary care. So it seems appropriate

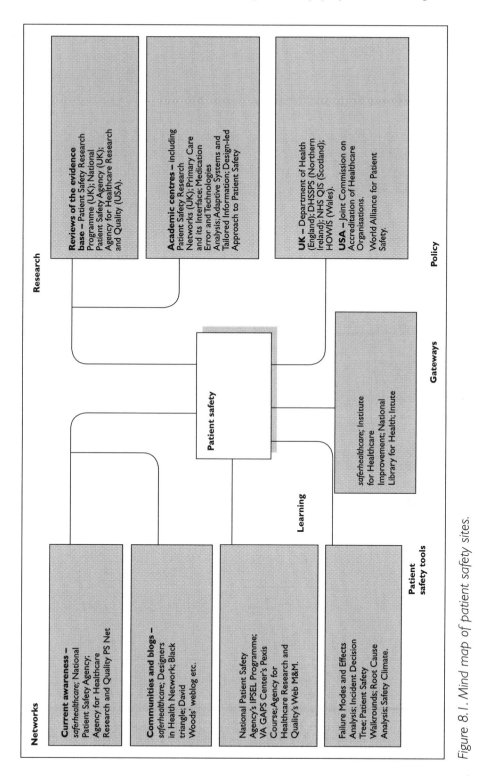

Figure 8.1. Mind map of patient safety sites.

that we begin the journey around our mind map of patient safety resources with a closer look at research in this area.

Research into Patient Safety

One of the most important collections of research in the UK is the Department of Health's (DH) *Patient Safety Research Programme*. The Director's Statement (Lilford, 2004) covers the genesis of the programme and its roots in government policy and its international links particularly with research in the US. The studies cover a wide range of topics including a review of the literature addressing communication in the context of error, lessons from litigation and error in primary care, in addition to studies focusing on responses to alerts about potassium chloride.

In the UK a number of other research networks have emerged. These include the *Patient Safety Research Network – Primary Care and its Interface*, based at the University of Manchester (University of Manchester, 2003), the *Medication Error and Technologies Analysis Network* (META) (University of London School of Pharmacy, 2003); the *Patient Safety Network — Adaptive Systems and Tailored Information* (University of Plymouth, 2003) and the design-led *Approach to Patient Safety Network* (University of Cambridge, 2003), among others. The *Clinical Safety and Research Unit* at Imperial College, London (2002) have published a review of the investigation and analysis of critical incidents and adverse events in healthcare that is available through the NHS *Health Technology Assessment Programme* (NHS, 2001).

The National Patient Safety Agency (NPSA) works in collaboration with the DH's Patient Safety Research Programme (PSRP), alongside others in the field in the UK and internationally. It too has published a strategy for its own programme of research (NPSA, 2004c). The NPSA is actively involved in other areas plotted on our map and we shall be dealing with its other activities including learning activities, and its mission to design and implement patient safety tools in the sections that follow.

In the US, the Agency for Healthcare Research and Quality (AHRQ) hosts one of the most important publicly available resources about patient safety. The *Medical Errors and Patient Safety* resource (Agency for Healthcare Research and Quality, 1999) contains key federally funded research such as *Making Health Care Safer: A Critical Analysis of Patient Safety Practices* (Agency for Healthcare Research and Quality, 2001), and provides up-to-date information on current research programmes. The AHRQ site is, however, much more than a repository of research and contains many other resources relating to other branches of our patient safety map. It produces the *Patient Safety E-Newsletter*

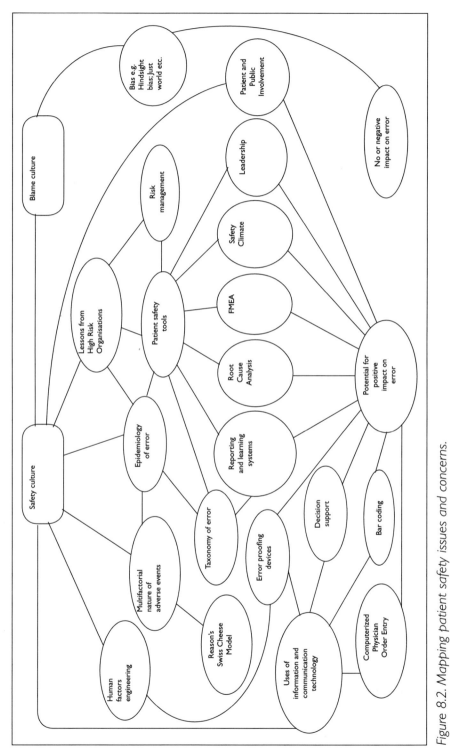

Figure 8.2. Mapping patient safety issues and concerns.

(Agency for Healthcare Research and Quality, 2004) and features *PS Net* (Agency for Healthcare Research and Quality, 2005), which is a continuously updated, annotated, and carefully selected collection of patient safety news, literature, tools, and resources.

Policy

In the UK, government policy on patient safety issues can be tracked online and many of the main policy documents in this area are available as pdf documents (DH, 2001; NHS QIS, 2005; Health of Wales Information Service, 2003). '*An Organisation with a Memory*' (DH, 2000) and '*Building a Safer NHS for patients*' (Smith, 2004) are important milestones. Equally significant is the archive of the inquiry into the Bristol Royal Infirmary (BRI) case, a watershed for public attitudes toward patient safety in the UK, and a catalyst government action (Kennedy, 2001).

The appearance of patient safety standards within recent policy documents from each of the four countries is testament to the impact of such widely reported systems failures (DH, 2004; Department of Health, Social Services and Public Safety, 2005; NHS QIS, 2005; Welsh Assembly Government, 2005). Risk management standards are an important corollary of these. In England the NHS Litigation Authority assesses member NHS bodies against a set of risk management standards that have been developed to reflect issues that consistently arise in negligence claims (NHS Litigation Authority, 2006).

The concentration of effort around safer healthcare practice is not confined to the UK. In fact, the phenomenon is global. In the USA the publication of '*To Err is Human: Building a Safer Health System*' (Institute of Medicine, 2000) heralded the arrival of a seismic shift in US healthcare policy.

In 2005, the Joint Commission on Accreditation of Healthcare Organizations and Joint Commission Resources announced the establishment of the Joint Commission International Center for Patient Safety (JCI Center for Patient Safety, 2005). The Joint Commission sets standards and evaluates the quality and safety of care for more than 15,000 health care organizations in the US. It promotes the delivery of safe, high-quality care through its *Sentinel Event Resource Index* (JCAHO, 2005b), *Sentinel Event Alert* (JCAHO, 2005a), *Speak Up*™ initiatives (JCAHO, 2002) and *National Patient Safety Goals* (JCAHO, 2006). The Patient Safety Center allows the Joint Commission to broaden the focus of its patient safety work including principles related to system design and organizational re-engineering, product safety, safety of services, and environment of care, as well as offering proactive solutions for patient safety, whether based on empirical evidence, hard research or best practices.

The same effect can be seen in many other countries around the world.

A list of international resources can be found at the National Patient Safety Foundation site (US). The list includes agencies in other countries such as the Australian Council for Safety and Quality in Health Care and other independent bodies, such as the Australian Patient Safety Foundation and the Canadian Patient Safety Institute.

Lately the effect on policy has entered a different stage with the recognition that co-ordinated efforts might have a greater impact. The World Health Organisation and key partners launched the World Alliance for Patient Safety in 2004. It aims to support the development of global norms and standards, encourage research and adoption of evidence-based policies (World Alliance for Patient Safety, 2004).

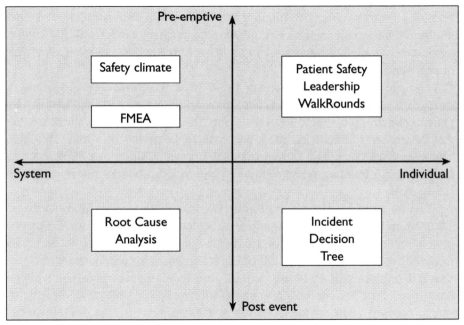

Figure 8.3 Contexts in which patient safety tools are used.
(FMEA=Failure Modes and Effects Analysis.)

Gateways

The energy flowing into the field of patient safety is being managed online, in some part, by the creation of subject area gateways. Some of these are called libraries, such as the National Library for Health (2005a) and the NHS Scotland e-Library (2005), and are similarly broad in their scope and collections. Healthcare gateways such as the health and life sciences area of the Intute are also a valuable part of the online landscape in that they support collections of valued and revised web-based resources contributed by information specialists. Others, for example *Saferhealthcare* (2005a), have a particular focus on the subject.

Like the AHRQ mentioned earlier, *Saferhealthcare* aims to be something of a one-stop shop for those with an active interest in the subject and much more than a repository of peer-reviewed articles. *Saferhealthcare* is an online patient safety resource and an opportunity for people interested this area to link up, share ideas and develop communities of interest. The website is a partnership between the National Patient Safety Agency (NPSA), BMJ Publishing Group, and the Institute for Healthcare Improvement. The community of practice idea is an integral part of the site. By registering with the resource you in effect become part of the collective intelligence of the site, with the ability to take part in discussions, receive newsletters, share patient safety stories and case studies, use interactive quality improvement tools over time and engage with a network of peers and subject experts.

The site is growing a library of topic areas which include such items as safety culture, medication practice, patient identification and discharging patients. Each topic area follows the same structure: a 'what we know' section that covers the literature on the topic; case studies; web sites and references. The site offers news and journal scan sections in addition to a products page highlighting e-learning resources, audio and video products and other patient safety tools.

The Institute for Healthcare Improvement is a partner in *Saferhealthcare*. The IHI is a not-for-profit organization specialising in developing practical implementation interventions for driving up quality. Founded in 1991 and based in Cambridge, Massachusetts, IHI offers comprehensive products and services. The IHI organises its resources around core topics of which patient safety is one. It also has influential programmes of work some of which are patient safety focused such as the *100k Lives Campaign* (Institute for Healthcare Improvement, 2005) which focused on avoidable deaths in hospitals.

Patient Safety Tools

One encouraging feature of the acute interest in patient safety is the urgency with which interventions have been tested and deployed. These patient safety tools are specifically designed to tackle different aspects of patient safety. *Figure 8.3* shows the context in which these tools are used:

If we follow the diagram clockwise, starting in the upper left quadrant, patient safety tools most often applied in an effort to effect changes in system pre-emptively include safety climate surveys (IHI, 2003) and Failure Modes and Effects Analysis (FMEA) (IHI, 2002b). The safety climate survey featured on the IHI website, was originally developed by the University of Texas. By using the survey tool an organization can gain information about the perceptions of front-line clinical staff about safety in their clinical area and management's commitment to safety. The survey also provides information about how perceptions vary across different departments and disciplines. By re-surveying over a period of time an organization can also monitor the impact of other initiatives that may have been introduced.

FMEA was originally developed for use in high-risk industries and has only been applied to healthcare relatively recently. FMEA is a systematic, proactive method for evaluating a process. Its purpose is to identify where and how the process might fail and to assess the relative impact of different failures, in order to identify the parts of the process that are most in need of change. The method looks at what could go wrong, why would the failure happen and what would be the consequences of such a failure. The IHI site includes additional information on related matters such as the meaning of Risk Priority Numbers and core processes in the ordering, dispensing and administering of medications.

In the upper right quadrant of *Figure 8.3,* Patient Safety Leadership WalkRounds (2002a) have been used to capture individual responses to issues as close as possible to the workplace before they escalate and lead to safety incidents. Patient Safety Leadership WalkRounds were promoted by the IHI as a means for leaders to establish a visible commitment to patient safety in their organisations. The IHI documentation describes their format and includes suggestions about questions for leaders to ask staff, which senior leaders should participate, and where to conduct them.

In the lower right quadrant Incident Decision Tree (*Saferhealthcare*, 2005b) are to support fairer decision-making when dealing with individuals at the sharp end of a patient safety incident. The Incident Decision Tree is being developed by the NPSA. It was specifically created to help NHS managers and senior clinicians decide whether they need to suspend (exclude) staff involved in a serious patient safety incident and to identify appropriate management action. The aim is to promote fair and consistent staff treatment within and between healthcare organisations. While the first pilot phase was tested in secondary care, the tool has now been extended to cover primary care organisations, general practices and community pharmacies.

In the lower left quadrant, Root Cause Analysis is promoted as a systematic way of gathering evidence following an incident in order to examine the contributing factors. The analysis is then used to identify areas for change, make recommendations and suggest sustainable solutions. The object is to encourage organisational learning in order to help minimise the re-occurrence of the incident type in the future.

The Root Cause Analysis (RCA) e-learning programme is a modular online training programme with support materials available to download and use (National Patient Safety Agency, 2003). The programme has been designed to help busy NHS staff whose training must adapt to fit hectic schedules. The learning programme describes a structured framework and a range of tools and techniques for the investigation and analysis of patient safety incidents. Divided into six modules, the first four provide an overview of RCA for those who need to undertake an RCA of a patient safety incident. The last two modules are more specialised for anyone wanting to obtain a deeper understanding of the theory behind RCA.

One of the often cited keys to nurturing a safety culture is establishing a system of reporting and learning from error. The National Patient Safety Agency is responsible for developing and co-ordinating the National Reporting and Learning System (2004a). The NPSA is encouraging the reporting of 'near misses', that is incidents that caused no harm to patients, or where harm was prevented, as well as events with a serious outcome, which are more likely to be flagged up in existing incident reporting systems. It is these prevented patient safety incidents that can provide the most valuable learning for the NHS, because they signal problem areas where there is potential for things to go wrong in the future. They can also highlight ways in which staff have prevented the incident harming the patient (or have minimised the actual harm caused to the patient), and the NPSA is looking to learn from these actions to encourage the spread of good practice. The NPSA is also developing a version of the electronic reporting form for the public and relevant third parties such as the NHS Patient Advice and Liaison Services (PALS) (2005b).

The IHI patient safety section has many other tools that may be of interest.

Learning

A number of free learning resources are available that provide important overviews of the topic. The Introduction to Patient Safety E-Learning Programme (IPSEL) from the NPSA has been designed specifically for NHS employees (NPSA, 2004b). The modules within IPSEL cover: an introduction to patient safety; guidance and support; reporting; patient safety solutions; team working; infusion devices; and misidentification.

Two notable web resources from the US are the Veteran's Administration GAPS Center (2002a) and AHRQ's Web M&M (Morbidity and Mortality Rounds on the WEB) (2003). The VA GAPS Center is a partnership of clinicians and experts in human performance funded to improve patient safety in healthcare. Two features of the site are useful in the context of learning materials. One section uses stories to provide engaging narratives that give concrete expression of fundamental patient safety concepts. The stories presented are from a variety of disciplines each story connects to a series of slides, a human factors explanation of the concept, provocative questions, and linked relevant websites. Healthcare patient safety stories include a wrong site surgery episode and a story about the introduction of a new paralyzing agent that demonstrates how a combination of latent failures occurring simultaneously created the conditions for an accident. The healthcare stories are counterbalanced by a selection from a range of other contexts.

The VA GAPS Center is also the home of the Pexis Course (2002b). The Pexis course also uses stories about disasters to teach concepts relating to predictable sources of systems failures within healthcare as well as in other complex industries as an introduction to examining the role of human factors in patient safety. .

AHRQ's Web M&M is described as an 'online journal and forum on patient safety and health care quality'. Readers can send in errors anonymously and have these commented on by experts. Interactive learning is present through 'spotlight cases'. Again these provide descriptions of actual cases and detailed analyses that draw out the implications for practice. For example, one case study features the story of a nurse preparing a patient in ICU for a CT scan. The nurse, rather than giving the contrast orally via a nasogastric tube (the appropriate route), infused the contrast solution intravenously. The subsequent commentary, by a nurse, explores the implications of 'floating' staff, issues around acknowledging error and the contribution of hospital leadership to a safety culture.

Communities and Blogs

The web has facilitated the development of a range of channels for exchanging news, publications and opinions on every conceivable topic. This is now reflected in the number of ways patient safety items can be published, exchanged and discussed. Some patient safety networks are academic, whilst others are more inclusive. The rise of blogging — writing an online journal or weblog (hence blog), has added a further method of web publishing (Wikipedia, 2005a).

We have already mentioned the cluster of research networks that have recently emerged in the UK under the research section. The Designers in Health Network runs a mailing list that can be joined via their website.

The National Academic Mailing List Service, known as 'JISCmail' (2005) manages a number of lists that might be of interest. The User Involvement Research mailing list (JISCmail, 2002) aims to 'bring together people with expertise in user involvement and public participation in the evaluation and delivery of public services'.

The UK based site *Saferhealthcare* incorporates a 'communities' area that invites users, once they have completed a free registration, to 'connect with peers, experts and future collaborators from around the world who have similar professions, organisational systems and interests'.

While many people might be reluctant to navigate through the 'blogosphere', blogs can provide interesting perspectives, especially when maintained by professionals working in the patient safety field. For instance, some blogs are written by academics.

If you want to track down blogs there are a number of ways to do it. Such is the popularity of blogging in the last few years a number of tools are now available to find them. Blog trackers such as *Technorati* and social bookmarking sites like *Del.icio.us* both use tags to categorise blog content. Many search engines such as *Google*, and *Blog Search Engine* have developed blog search functions. Blog directories are also building lists of blogs by themes or topics. When you have found a blog you like it is worth checking the blogroll, or list of other recommended blogs, you are likely to find there.

Current Awareness

Patient safety is a multifaceted topic and the subject of intense global debate. One by-product of this interest from a healthcare perspective is the utilisation of the web as a channel for dissemination. The NPSA, for example, publishes advice on topics in various formats: Patient Safety Alerts requiring prompt action to address high risk safety problems; Safer Practice Notices that strongly advise implementing particular recommendations or solutions, and Patient Safety Information that suggest issues or effective techniques that healthcare staff might consider to enhance safety (NPSA, 2005a).

Registering with sites such as *Saferhealthcare* is a useful way maintaining current awareness through newsletters and email updates about the launch of new topics, features and content posted to the site.

Really Simple Syndication (RSS) is another addition to the ways in which web users can subscribe to services that alert them to items on issues of interest to them (Wikipedia, 2005b). Many virtual libraries like the National Library for Health are developing news and RSS areas (2005b).

References

AHRQ (1999) *Medical Errors and Patient Safety*. http://www.ahrq.gov/qual/errorsix. htm (accessed 22nd January 2006)

AHRQ (2001) *Making Health Care Safer: A Critical Analysis of Patient Safety*

Practices. Evidence Report/Technology Assessment: Number 43. http://www.ahrq. gov/clinic/ptsafety/ (accessed 22nd January 2006)

AHRQ (2003) *WebM&M (Morbidity and Mortality Rounds on the WEB).* http://www. webmm.ahrq.gov (accessed 22nd January 2006)

AHRQ (2004) *Patient Safety E-Newsletter Archives.* http://www.ahrq.gov/news/ ptsnews.htm (accessed 22nd January 2006)

AHRQ (2005) PSNet. http://psnet.ahrq.gov/index.aspx (accessed 22nd January 2006).

Buzan T, Buzan B (2006) *The Mind Map Book.* BBC Active, London

Cohen J, Stewart I (1997) *Figments of reality. The evolution of the curious mind.* Cambridge University Press, Cambridge

Dale A (2003) *Information – it's all in the mind.* http://www.cilip.org.uk/publications/ updatemagazine/archive/archive2003/april/update0304b.htm (accessed 22nd January 2006)

DH (2001) *Patient safety.* http://www.dh.gov.uk/PolicyAndGuidance/ HealthAndSocialCareTopics/PatientSafety/fs/en (accessed 22nd January 2006)

DH (2004) *Standards for Better Health.* http://www.dh.gov.uk/ assetRoot/04/08/66/66/04086666.pdf (accessed 22nd January 2006)

DH (2000) *An Organisation with a Memory.* The Stationary Office, London. (accessed 22nd January 2006)

Department of Health, Social Services and Public Safety (2005) *Best Practice, Best Care: The Quality Standards for Health and Social Care.* http://www.dhsspsni. gov.uk/hss/governance/quality_standards.asp (accessed 22nd January 2006)

Designers in Health Network (1996) *DiHNet.* http://www.dihnet.org.uk/ (accessed 22nd January 2006)

Imperial College London (2002). *Clinical Safety Research Unit* http://www.csru.org. uk/ (accessed 22nd January 2006)

Institute for Healthcare Improvement (2002b) *Failure Modes and Effects Analysis.* http://www.ihi.org/IHI/Topics/PatientSafety/SafetyGeneral/Tools/Failure+Modes +and+Effects+Analysis+%28FMEA%29+Tool+%28IHI+Tool%29.htm (accessed 22nd January 2006)

Institute for Healthcare Improvement (2003) *Safety Climate Survey.* http://www.ihi. org/IHI/Topics/PatientSafety/MedicationSystems/Tools/Safety+Climate+Survey+(IHI+Tool).htm (accessed 22nd January 2006)

Institute for Healthcare Improvement (2005) *100k Lives Campaign.* http://www.ihi. org/IHI/Programs/Campaign/ (accessed 22nd January 2006).

Institute of Medicine (2000) *To err is human: Building a Safer Health System. National* Academy Press, Washington DC

Intute (2006) *Health and life sciences.* https://intute.ac.uk/healthandlifesciences (accessed 13 July 2006)

JCAHO (2002) *Speak Up Initiatives.* http://www.jcaho.org/accredited+organizations/ speak+up/index.htm (accessed 22nd January 2006)

JCAHO (2005a) *Sentinel Event Alert*. http://www.jcaho.org/about+us/news+letters/sentinel+event+alert/ (accessed 22nd January 2006)

JCAHO (2005b) *Sentinel Event Resource Index*. http://www.jcaho.org/accredited+organizations/sentinel+event/se_index.htm (accessed 22nd January 2006)

JCAHO (2006) *National Patient Safety Goals*. http://www.jcaho.org/accredited+organizations/patient+safety/npsg.htm (accessed 22nd January 2006)

JISCmail (2002) T*he User Involvement Research mailing list*. http://www.jiscmail.ac.uk/lists/USER-INVOLVEMENT.html (accessed 22nd January 2006)

Kennedy I (2001) T*he Report of the Public Inquiry into Children's Heart Surgery at the Bristol Royal Infirmary 1984-1995*. Stationery Office, London

Lilford R (2004) *The Director's Statement*. Patient Safety Research Programme in England and Wales, Department of Public Health and Epidemiology, University of Birmingham. http://www.pcpoh.bham.ac.uk/publichealth/psrp/Pdf/Directors_Statement.pdf (accessed 22nd January 2006)

National Library for Health (2005b) *News & RSS*. http://www.library.nhs.uk/rss/ (accessed 22nd January 2006)

National Patient Safety Agency (2003) *Root Cause Analysis Training*. http://www.npsa.nhs.uk/health/resources/root_cause_analysis/conditions

National Patient Safety Agency (2004a) *National Reporting and Learning System* http://www.npsa.nhs.uk/health/reporting/background (accessed 22nd January 2006)

National Patient Safety Agency (2004b) *Introduction to Patient Safety E-Learning Programme (IPSEL)*. http://www.npsa.nhs.uk/health/resources/ipsel (accessed 22nd January 2006)

National Patient Safety Agency (2004c). *Research and Development Strategy*. http://www.npsa.nhs.uk/site/media/documents/1279_NPSA_R&D_Strategy.pdf (accessed 22nd January 2006)

National Patient Safety Agency (2005a) *A summary of NPSA's dissemination processes*. http://www.npsa.nhs.uk/web/display?contentId=3092 (accessed 22nd January 2006)

NHS Litigation Authority (2006) Risk Management Publications. Standards.https://www.nhsla.com/Publications (accessed 22 January 2006)

NHS QIS (2005) *Clinical Governance and Risk Management: Achieving Safe, Effective, Patient-focused Care and Services*. NHS Scotland. http://www.nhshealthquality.org/nhsqis/files/CGRM_CSF_Oct05.pdf (accessed 22nd January 2006)

Saferhealthcare (2005b) *Incident Decision Tree*. http://www.saferhealthcare.org.uk/IHI/Products/OtherProducts/idt2.htm (accessed 22nd January 2006).

Saferhealthcare (2005c) *Discussion groups*. http://www.saferhealthcare.org.uk/ihi/community/ (accessed 22nd January 2006)

Saferhealthcare (no date) *Root Cause Analysis Toolkit*. http://www.saferhealthcare.

org.uk/IHI/Products/E-learning/rcatoolkit.htm (accessed 22nd January 2006).

Scrivener R (2002) *Mapping health on the Internet. Strategies for learning in an information age*. Radcliffe Medical Press, Abingdon

Smith J (2004) *Building a safer NHS for patients. Improving Medication Safety*. The Stationary Office, London

University of Birmingham (2002) *Patient Safety Research Programme*. http://www. pcpoh.bham.ac.uk/publichealth/psrp/ (accessed 22nd January 2006)

University of Cambridge (2003) *Design-led approach to patient safety*. http://www-edc.eng.cam.ac.uk/medical/ (accessed 22nd January 2006)

University of London (2003) *Patient Safety Network – Medication Error and Technologies Analysis*. http://www.meta-network.org/ (accessed 22nd January 2006)

University of Manchester (2003) *Patient Safety Network – Primary Care and its Interface*. http://www.ihs.man.ac.uk/PSRN (accessed 22nd January 2006).

University of Plymouth (2003) *Patient Safety Network – Adaptive Systems and Tailored Inforation*. http://www.patientsafetynetwork.psy.plymouth.ac.uk/ (accessed 22nd January 2006).

Veterans Administration GAPS Center (2002b) *Pexis Course*. http://csel.eng.ohio-state.edu/productions/pexis/index.html (accessed 22nd January 2006)

Welsh Assembly Government (2005) *Healthcare Standards for Wales. Making the Connections. Designed for Life. NHS Wales*. http://www.wales.gov.uk/subihealth/ content/keypubs/pdf/healthcare-standards-e.pdf (accessed 22nd January 2006)

Wikipedia (2005a) http://en.wikipedia.org/wiki/Blog (accessed 22 January 2006)

Wikipedia (2005b) http://en.wikipedia.org/wiki/Rss (accessed 22 January 2006)

Resources

Australian Patient Safety Foundation: http://www.apsf.net.au

Blog Search Engine: http://www.blogsearchengine.com

Bristol Royal Infirmary Inquiry: http://www.bristol-inquiry.org.uk

Britblog.com: http://www.britblog.com

Canadian Patient Safety Institute: http://www.patientsafetyinstitute.ca/index.html

Del.icio.us: http://del.icio.us.co.uk

Department of Health, Social Services and Public Safety: http://www.dhsspsni.gov. uk/index.asp

Health of Wales Information Service: http://www.wales.nhs.uk

Institute for Healthcare Improvement: http://www.ihi.org

Intute: https://www.intute.ac.uk

National Library for Health: http://www.library.nhs.uk

National Patient Safety Agency: http://www.npsa.nhs.uk/ppr

National Patient Safety Foundation: http://www.npsf.org

NHS Health Technology Assessment Programme: http://www.hta.nhsweb.nhs.uk

NHS Litigation Authority: http://www.nhsla.com

NHS Quality Improvement Scotland: http://www.nhshealthquality.org

NHS Scotland e-Library: (http://www.elib.scot.nhs.uk/portal/elib/pages/index.aspx

NMAP: http://nmap.ac.uk

OMNI: http://omni.ac.uk

Saferhealthcare: http://www.saferhealthcare.org.uk/ihi

Technorati: http://www.technorati.com

Veterans Administration GAPS Center: http://www.gapscenter.org/Stories.asp

World Alliance for Patient Safety: http://www.who.int/patientsafety/worldalliance/en

Index